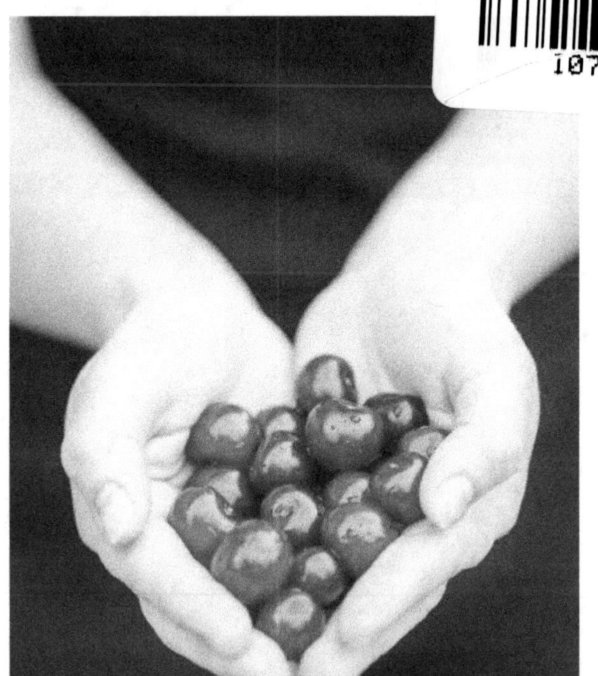

Dash Diet Cookbook

15-Day Meal Plan - Simple, Quick & Tasty Recipes to
Help Treat Hypertension & Lose Weight

By Silvia Pala

Table of Contents

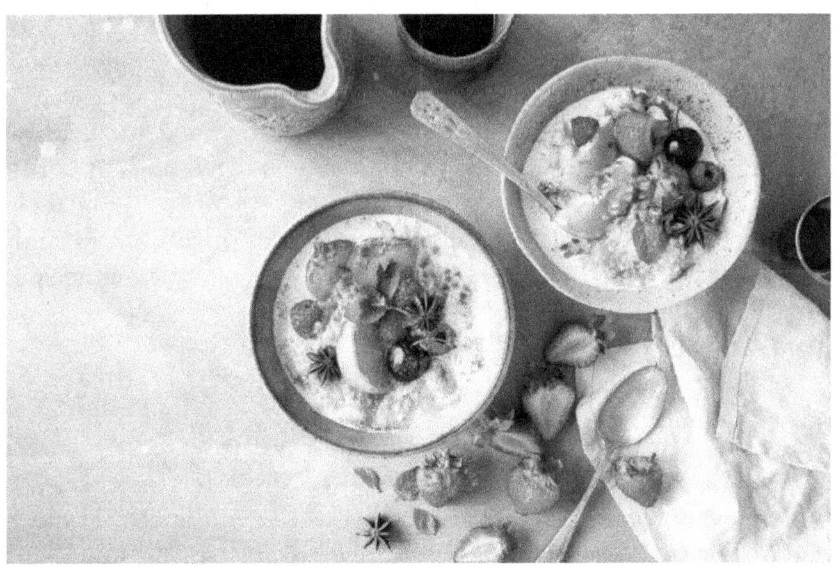

Introduction

I would like to offer you a dash of salt and a dash of pepper to introduce you to the DASH Diet *(Dietary Approaches to Stop Hypertension)*. This healthy approach includes food *(and drinks)* that help treat hypertension in just two weeks!

This healthy eating approach will show you how in 2 weeks you can help prevent or treat your hypertension and other unhealthy blood pressure issues and improve your overall health.

The ultimate goal of the DASH diet is to offer a variety of healthy foods in appropriate servings. The DASH way of eating will help your body get the most out of proper daily nutrition. This diet brings the following benefits:

- ✔ Help reduce the risk of stroke, heart disease, and heart failure
- ✔ Aid in losing weight/ promotes health-conscious weight loss
- ✔ Help reduce the risk of developing *(various types of)* diabetes
- ✔ Help prevent the formation of kidney stones; it slows down the development of *(various types of)* kidney disease
- ✔ Help reduce the risk of Polycystic ovary syndrome (PCOS) or postmenopausal weight gain

✔ Help lower LDL cholesterol levels
✔ Help relieve depression

This healthy diet approach is highly recommended for people suffering from hypertension *(high blood pressure)* and/or pre-hypertension.

Don't like vegetables? Don't worry. Both meat lovers and vegetarians will find the DASH Diet very easy to follow. Each recipe in our 2-week plan holds true to the following:

✔ All natural
✔ No preservatives
✔ No additives
✔ Unprocessed

Now, what food and beverages can you have in the DASH diet? Read on for more valuable information about this amazing diet!

What was your motivation for selecting this book? Please let me know your feedback and thoughts by **_leaving a review on Amazon_**, *because this 'open' way of communicating may help others who have read the book or are interested in reading it.*

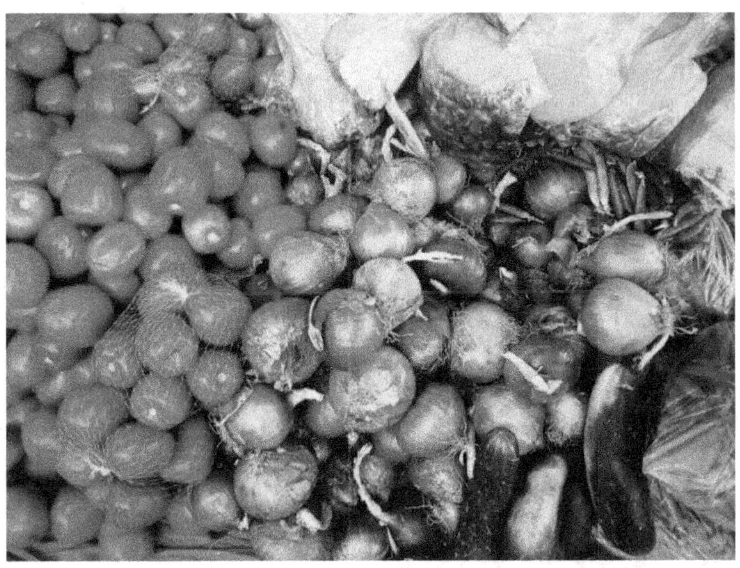

Chapter 1 – A Dash of Healthy Diet: The DASH Diet

Have you heard of The DASH diet? It simply contains a dash of nutritiously healthy things! NOT a dash of unhealthy ingredients is included in this diet plan. Read on for more valuable information about The DASH Diet.

What is the DASH Diet?

The DASH Diet is an acronym for Dietary Approaches to Stop Hypertension. The DASH Diet includes deliciously healthy foods *(and even drinks)* rich in plant-based ingredients and paired with protein-rich meat.

The DASH diet program was created by a panel of health experts at the National Institutes of Health (NIH) in the early 1990s. Its main purpose is to help people lower their blood pressure by changing their eating lifestyle. Two experimental DASH diet plans were curated and carried out as a randomized, outpatient feeding trial to test the effects of nutritional eating patterns on blood pressure. The unique feature of the experimental DASH diet program is that its menu was based on foods usually consumed, so people could easily adapt to it.

The initial DASH diet studies have proven to the world its effectiveness in reducing excess fats while being healthy at the same time. It has shown that taking more than 3,000 milligrams of sodium per day can actually tame high blood pressure, as well as its first line blood pressure values! This diet approach proves you can help reduce hypertension even if you are putting more than a dash of salt on your everyday dishes!

The original DASH diet studies were high in starchy ingredients and refined grains.

The DASH diet studies found out that on average, the dieters' blood pressure dropped by 6.7 mmHg in systolic phase and 3.5 mmHg in diastolic phase in 2 weeks *(with negligible side effects)*.

Advantages of the DASH Diet

The DASH Diet plan is exclusively designed to provide substantial amounts of key nutrients that target hypertension. It is a sustainable eating plan for a healthy lifestyle based on nutritious foods. Below are the advantages of the DASH diet plan:

- **Proven Effective** – The DASH diet plan brings bountiful benefits in help treating hypertension and various diseases. Eating the DASH way dramatically helps reduce high blood pressure, excess body fats, LDL cholesterol, triglycerides, and much more!

- **Good Whole Foods** – The DASH diet encourages its followers to eat only whole superfoods.

- **Nutritiously Good** – The DASH diet plan is designed to guide you to eat only the most nutrient-dense food and beverages. It dashes you away from consuming empty calories and highly-processed foods, so you lose weight easily without feeling hungry.

- **Cost-effective** – The food, drinks and ingredients included in the DASH diet plan are not expensive. DASH doesn't require buying food supplements, dietary supplements, etc..

- **Adjustable Diet Plan** – With the DASH diet, it is easy to adjust the levels of nutritional content per serving. For instance, you can adjust calorie levels from 1,200, 1,600,

2,000, 2,500, 3,000 mg per serving, etc. You can easily adapt to your body's preferred level, adjusting them as you transition to a lifelong healthy eating pattern.

Disadvantages of the DASH Diet

Even dietary plans come with disadvantages, but these have nothing to do with health. Below are the disadvantages of the DASH diet plan:

- **Not Easily Accessible** – Since the DASH diet plan is not a commercialized eating program, pre-packed and/or precooked foods and store-bought beverages are strictly not allowed. That is, you cannot go to the freezer section of the market and buy frozen goodies. The Dietary Approaches to Stop Hypertension requires work.
- **Strictly Portioned Servings** – For best results, the DASH diet's strictly portioned servings need to be carefully planned. You must always keep track of the servings from each and every dish or drink that you consume.
- **Being Aware of Food Labels** – When you follow the DASH diet, we highly advise making it a habit to read food labels carefully. You must check any hidden sources of sugar, sodium, food additives, preservatives, etc. in the ingredients that you buy.
- **Not Travel-Friendly** – Traveling and eating outside your house can be difficult, as you do not know how the food is cooked. You won't be sure whether you are eating whole and natural food and beverages. To play it safe, look for a restaurant that offers organic food and beverages.
- **Bland Food and Beverages** – If you have suddenly decided to follow the DASH diet or transition to a healthy eating lifestyle, it may take you time to get used to food and beverages with less flavor.

What to Eat

The Dietary Approaches to Stop Hypertension, widely known as the DASH diet, encourages you to strictly eat (and drink) the following:

✔ **Fruits** – Includes apple, pear, peach, all types of berries, and tropical fruits such as pineapple, mango, etc. *(about 4-5 servings per day)*

✔ **Green, Leafy Vegetables** – Includes cauliflower, broccoli, cabbage, spinach, green beans, dry beans, kale, etc. *(about 4-5 servings per day)*

✔ **Lean Protein Meat and Fish** – Includes poultry, beans, and seafood *(fewer than 6 servings per day)*

✔ **Whole Grain** – Includes bread, pasta, rice, and cereal *(about 6-8 servings per day)*

✔ **Fat-Free or Low-Fat Condiments** – Includes skim milk, cheese, and yogurt *(2-3 servings per day)*

✔ **Nuts, Legumes, and Seeds** – Includes peanuts, hazelnuts, walnuts, sunflower seeds, flax seeds, watermelon seeds, split peas, kidney beans, lentils, etc. *(3-5 servings per week)*

✔ **Heart-Healthy Cooking Oils** – Includes vegetable, canola, olive, safflower, and corn oils; low-fat mayonnaise; light salad dressing; butter, and margarine *(2-3 servings per day)*

✔ **Healthy Sugar Substitutes/ Wholesome Sweeteners** – Includes agave nectar, muscovado sugar, etc. *(fewer than 5 servings per day)*

✔ **Low-Calorie Beverages** – Includes water, flavored water, and tea. Drinking coffee on the DASH diet is still debatable.

✔ **Unsalted Snacks** – Snacks in the DASH diet are all unsalted *(but not bland, because the ingredients used in the DASH snacks are naturally and nutritiously salty)*

✔ **Unsweetened Desserts** – Desserts in the DASH diet are all unsweetened *(but not bland, because the ingredients used in the DASH desserts are naturally and nutritiously sweet)*

What NOT to Eat

The DASH diet plan restricts the following:

- **Sodium** – The DASH diet strictly recommends consume at least 1,500 mg *(3/4 teaspoon)* and not more than 2,300 mg of sodium per day *(1 teaspoon)*.
- **Added Sugar and other Sweeteners** – Includes table sugar, candies, soft drinks and/or sugar-loaded beverages, unrefined sugar, etc.
- **Bad Fat** – Includes saturated fat, trans-fat, LDL cholesterol, etc.
- **Caffeinated Products** – It is still being debated whether to include these as part of the DASH diet. Caffeinated products can cause a slight rise in blood pressure (BP) of about 5-10 mmHg. DASH dieters who have normal BP are recommended to drink 3-4 regular coffees per day.
- **Alcoholic Beverages** – A healthy lifestyle usually does not include alcoholic beverages. Alcohol could cause high blood pressure.
- **Unhealthy Cooking Oils** – Includes coconut oil and palm oil.
- **Red Meat** – Eating red meat could worsen high blood pressure, since this type of meat is high in saturated fats and LDL cholesterol.
- **Fatty Meat** – Whenever you buy meat, always trim off the fatty parts; these include bad cholesterol that will worsen your hypertension.
- **Full-Fat Dairy** – As the name implies, dairy that is full of fat contributes to excess fats in the human body.
- **Refined Grains** – Refined grains are not the same as whole grain. Refined grains could contribute to abdominal fats (and other excess fats in the human body), various kinds of heart diseases and different types of diabetes.

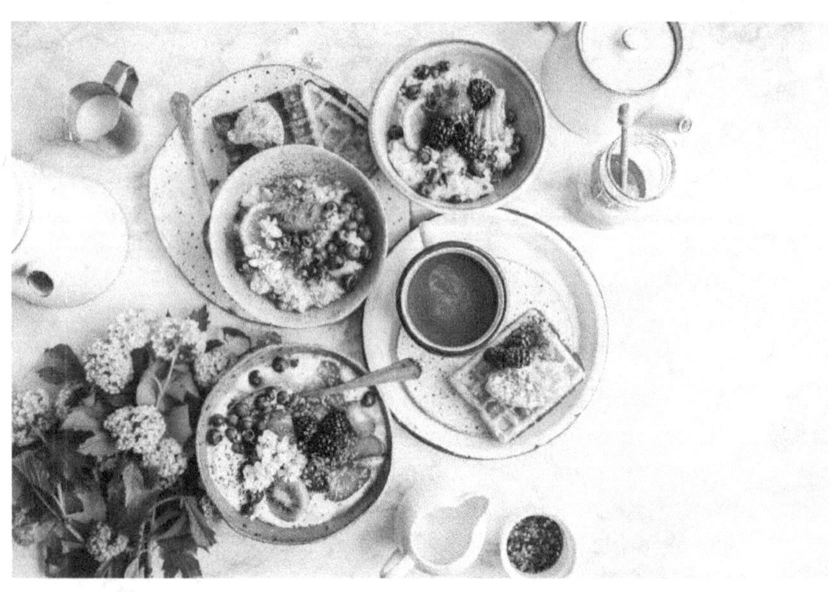

Chapter 2 – The 2-Week DASH Diet Plan

Now that you know the food and beverages that are included *(and not included)*, we have carefully curated a 2-week DASH diet plan just for you!

DASH Diet Plan	Breakfast	Appetizer	Main Course	Dessert	Dinner
Day 1	Berry Honey Overnight Oats	Chicken Quesadillas	Baked Chicken with Onion, Tarragon, and Wild Rice	Poached Pears	Black Beans and Sweet Potato Rice Bowl
Day 2	Banana Nutty Oats	Italian Sausage Zucchini Boats	Beefy Veggie Soup	Pumpkin with Chia Seeds Pudding	DASH Cannellini Corn Pasta

Day 3	Cherry Cocoa Oats	Cherry-Chicken Lettuce Cups	Strawberry Blue Cheese Steak	DASH Chocolate Truffles	Orange and Pistachio-Crusted Pork Tenderloin with Rice
Day 4	Carrot Overnight Oats	Turkey Barbecue Burger	Poached Salmon Miso	Grilled Pineapple Strips	Chickpea Curry
Day 5	Banana Colada Oats	Sweet Potato and Chickpea Pita Doner	Seared Chicken with Mango Salsa	Raspberry Peach Pancake	Fried Chicken with Cauliflower Rice Bowl
Day 6	Portobello Mushroom and Sausage Florentine	Sesame Chicken Veggie Tortilla Wraps	Barbecue Pork Chops with Roasted Spinach and Kale	Mango Rice Pudding	Garlic-Roasted Salmon with Brussel Sprouts
Day 7	Asparagus Omelet	Lime Chicken Tacos	Orange Sesame Shrimp	Choco Banana Cake	Pork Curry with Rice Noodles
Day 8	Salsa Frittata	Black Bean Burger	Creamy Chicken Pasta	Zesty Zucchini Muffins	Spiced Turkey in Lettuce Cups
Day 9	Berry Banana Brunch	Tomato and Basil Bruschetta	DASH Meaty Spaghetti	Blueberry Oats Muffins	Noodle-Less Lasagna
Day 10	Slow Cooker Apple Cinnamon Oatmeal	Artichoke Hearts Spinach Dip	Pork Chop Curry with Roasted Apples and Leeks	DASH Banana Bread	DASH Chicken Piccata

Day 11	Buckwheat Crepes	Chicken Enchiladas	Roasted Pork Tenderloin with Rhubarb Barbecue Sauce	DASH Milk Chocolate Pudding	DASH Shepherd's Pie
Day 12	Sweet Potato Waffles	DASH Acorn Squash Rings	Tuna Melts	Minty Lime and Grapefruit Yogurt Parfait	DASH Roasted Turkey
Day 13	DASH French Toast	DASH Delicata Squash Rounds	Quinoa Meatless Balls	DASH Peach Tarts	DASH Mac and Cheese
Day 14	Tofu Egg Scramble	Cottage Cheese and Roasted Tomato Topped Potatoes	Quinoa Black Bean Burger	DASH Raspberry Nuts Parfait	Lime Tilapia Fillets
Day 15	Bella Mushroom and Spinach Omelet	Cheesy Broccoli Baked Potato Hams	Cranberry Chicken Bowl	Strawberry Bruschetta	Beef Stroganoff

Chapter 3 – A Dash of Bountiful Breakfast

Start your day right with a dash of bountiful breakfast. All recipes bring the best nutrients you need for the entire day.

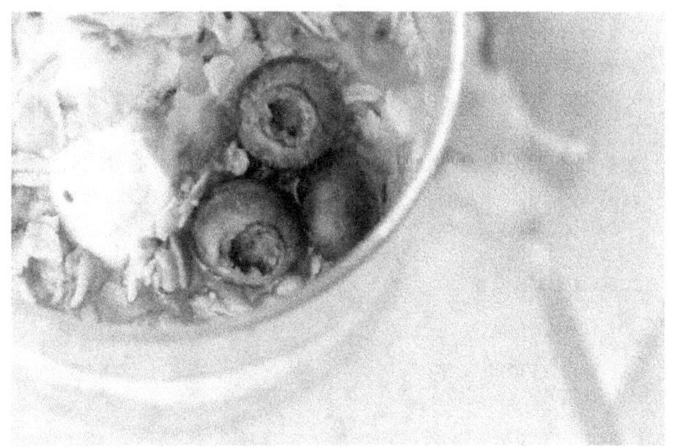

Berry Honey Overnight Oats

Preparation 10 minutes plus chilling time   *Servings* 1
Nutritional Information

Start your DASH diet plan with a "berry" sweet breakfast oatmeal. Overnight oats are prepared the night before, so you can get a bit of extra sleep in the morning.

Ingredients
½ cup fresh berries
1/3 cup oats
1 tablespoon raw honey
2 tablespoons vegetable oil
2 tablespoons walnuts, roughly chopped and toasted
3 tablespoons fat-free coconut milk
3 tablespoons plain, low-fat yogurt

Preparation
1. Combine oats, honey, coconut milk, and yogurt in a jar or any small container.
2. Toast walnuts; heat vegetable oil to cook walnuts on low heat till light brownish, stirring occasionally.

3. Top your berry honey overnight oats with berries and walnuts.
4. Cover the container tightly.
5. Refrigerate overnight and serve chilled in the morning.

Nutritional Information	Per Serving
Sodium	53 milligrams
Calories	345 milligrams
Fats	13 grams
Saturated Fats	2 grams
Cholesterol	4 milligrams
Carbohydrates	53 grams
Fibers	5 grams
Proteins	10 grams

Banana Nutty Oats

Preparation 10 minutes plus chilling time   *Servings* 1

Nutritional Information

Bananas are free of fats, bad cholesterol and sodium, and are filled with vitamins and minerals to jump-start your day! Try this banana nutty oatmeal recipe for a DASH lifestyle.

Ingredients

½ teaspoon cinnamon
1/3 cup oats
1 piece of banana, chopped bite-sized
1 tablespoon maple syrup
2 tablespoons vegetable oil
2 tablespoons toasted pecans
3 tablespoons soy milk
3 tablespoons plain, low-fat yogurt

Preparation

1. Combine oats, banana bits, cinnamon, maple syrup, soy milk, and yogurt in a jar or any small container.
2. Toast pecans; heat vegetable oil to cook pecans on low heat till light brownish, stirring occasionally.
3. Top mixture with pecans and cover the container.
4. Refrigerate overnight and serve chilled in the morning.

Nutritional Information	Per Serving
Sodium	0 milligrams
Calories	183 milligrams
Fats	18 grams
Saturated Fats	1.7 grams
Cholesterol	4 milligrams
Carbohydrates	53 grams
Fibers	3 grams
Proteins	4 grams
Potassium	450 milligrams

Folates	25.0 micrograms
Magnesium	34 milligrams
Manganese	0.3 milligrams

Cherry Cocoa Oats

Preparation 10 minutes plus chilling time   *Servings* 1

Nutritional Information

Cherries are rich in proteins, iron, potassium, and vitamins A and C. Pair them with cocoa for a DASH of sweetness by following this recipe:

Ingredients

A handful of frozen, pitted cherries

1/3 cup oats

1 tablespoon cocoa powder

3 tablespoons low-fat milk

3 tablespoons plain, low-fat yogurt

Preparation

1. Combine oats, maple syrup, low-fat milk, and yogurt in a jar or any small container.
2. Top mixture with cherries and cover the container.
3. Refrigerate overnight and serve chilled in the morning.

Nutritional Information	Per Serving
Sodium	0 milligrams
Calories	21 milligrams
Fats	13 grams
Saturated Fats	0 grams
Total Fats	0.5 grams
Cholesterol	0 milligrams
Carbohydrates	3 grams
Fibers	5 grams
Proteins	10 grams
Potassium	260 milligrams

Carrot Overnight Oats

Preparation 10 minutes plus chilling time   *Servings* 1
Nutritional Information
Carrots are a good source of vitamins and minerals such as beta-carotene, biotin, potassium, vitamin A, K, and B6. Start your day the DASH way by following this simple recipe:

Ingredients
1/3 cup oats
2 tablespoons carrots, grated
3 tablespoons low-fat coconut milk
3 tablespoons cream cheese, low-fat

Preparation
1. Combine oats, grated carrots, low-fat milk, and cream cheese in a jar or any small container.
2. Cover the container.
3. Refrigerate overnight and serve chilled in the morning.

Nutritional Information	Per Serving
Sodium	69 milligrams
Calories	41 milligrams
Total Fats	0.2 grams
Saturated Fats	0 gram
Polyunsaturated Fats	0.1 gram
Monounsaturated Fats	0 gram
Trans Fats	0 gram
Cholesterol	0 milligrams
Potassium	320 milligrams
Total Carbohydrates	10 grams
Proteins	0.9 grams

Banana Colada Oats

Preparation 10 minutes plus chilling time   *Servings* 1
Nutritional Information
Bananas are rich in vitamins and minerals such as Vitamin B, while pineapples are a good source of dietary fibers, folates, manganese, pantothenic acid, and ascorbic acid. Here's how to make this unique cola-DASH recipe:

Ingredients
1/3 cup oats
1 banana, chopped bite-sized
1 tablespoon shredded coconut
2 tablespoons crushed pineapple
3 tablespoons low-fat coconut milk

Preparation
1. Combine oats, coconut milk, and crushed pineapple in a jar or any small container.
2. Top mixture with shredded coconut meat and banana bits.
3. Cover the container.
4. Refrigerate overnight and serve chilled in the morning.

Nutritional Information	Per Serving
Sodium	1 milligram
Calories	50 milligrams
Total Fats	0.1 gram
Cholesterol	0 milligram
Potassium	109 milligrams
Total Carbohydrates	13 grams
Proteins	0.5 grams

Portobello Mushroom and Sausage Florentine

Preparation 30 minutes   *Servings* 2
Nutritional Information
For a dash of a hearty breakfast to bring flavor to your mornings, try this easy recipe:

Ingredients
Vegetable oil cooking spray
One handful minced basil
½ teaspoon olive oil
¼ cup crumbled goat cheese
1/8 teaspoon garlic salt
1/8 teaspoon salt
1/8 teaspoon ground black pepper
1 small minced onion
1 small unprocessed sausage, chopped bite-sized
1 cup baby spinach, minced
2 large organic eggs
2 large Portobello mushrooms, stems trimmed

Preparation
1. Preheat oven to 425 °F
2. Spray Portobello mushrooms with vegetable oil; place stem-side-up on a baking pan lined with parchment paper; dash with garlic salt and ground black pepper.
3. Place the Portobello mushrooms in the oven and bake uncovered till tender for 15 minutes.
4. In a non-stick skillet, heat vegetable oil over medium heat to cook sausage and sauté onion until tender; add spinach and cook until wilted.
5. In a bowl, whisk eggs then add a dash of salt and pour the mixture in the skillet. Cook and stir the egg until the texture thickens.
6. Scoop the egg mixture into the Portobello mushrooms; sprinkle with goat cheese and basil.
7. Serve immediately.

Nutritional Information	Per Serving
Sodium	472 milligrams
Calories	126 milligrams
Total Fats	5 grams
Saturated Fats	2 grams
Cholesterol	18 milligrams
Carbohydrates	10 grams
Dietary Fibers	3 grams
Proteins	11 grams

Asparagus Omelet

Preparation 30 minutes   *Servings* 1
Nutritional Information
Asparagus is rich in folates, calcium, proteins, fibers, and iron. Wrap it in an omelet for an excellent source of disease-killing nutrients such as lutein, proteins, carotenoids, and much more!

Ingredients
1/8 teaspoon ground black pepper
1 tablespoon fat-free milk
1 teaspoon butter
1 minced green onion
2 large organic egg
2 tablespoons Parmesan grated cheese
4 asparagus spears, trimmed and chopped

Preparation
1. Whisk egg, milk, Parmesan cheese, and ground black pepper in a bowl.
2. Coat a non-stick skillet with butter, pour in half of the omelet mixture and cook over medium heat.
3. Add the asparagus; cook and stir frequently until crispy yet tender; remove from the pan.
4. As the omelet edges set, sprinkle the green onion.
5. Fold the omelet in half, then flip it to cook the other side.
6. Remove from heat, transfer to a platter, and serve immediately.

Nutritional Information	Per Serving
Sodium	444 milligrams
Calories	319 milligrams
Total Fats	13 grams
Saturated Fats	5 grams
Cholesterol	225 milligrams
Carbohydrates	28 grams
Dietary Fibers	3 grams

Salsa Frittata

Preparation 40 minutes   *Servings* 6
Nutritional Information
Black beans are an excellent source of fibers and proteins. This DASH version of Frittata is filled with nutritiously flavorful ingredients to pump up your mornings. Here's how to make it:

Ingredients
1/3 cup minced green pepper
1/3 cup minced red bell pepper
½ cup shredded white cheddar cheese
¼ cup homemade salsa
¼ teaspoon iodized salt
¼ teaspoon ground black pepper
1 tablespoon olive oil
1 tablespoon minced parsley
1 cup black beans, drained
2 minced garlic cloves
3 green onions, minced
6 large organic eggs

Preparation
1. Preheat broiler.
2. Whisk eggs, homemade salsa, parsley, iodized salt, ground black pepper, and olive oil in a bowl.
3. In an oven-proof skillet, heat olive oil over medium-high heat to sauté green onions and green/red bell peppers; cook and stir frequently for 5 minutes until tender; add garlic and cook for a minute until brownish and fragrant; stir in black beans and cook until heated through.
4. Pour the egg mixture, cook uncovered for 5 minutes until it is nearly set; sprinkle with white cheddar cheese.
5. Transfer to the broiler to broil for 5 minutes until the egg is light golden brown and completely cooked.
6. Allow to sit for a few minutes then slice into wedges.
7. Serve on a platter.

Nutritional Information	Per Serving
Sodium	378 milligrams
Calories	183 milligrams
Total Fats	10 grams
Saturated Fats	4 grams
Cholesterol	196 milligrams
Carbohydrates	9 grams
Dietary Fibers	2 grams
Proteins	13 grams

Berry Banana Brunch

Preparation 10 minutes   *Servings* 4

Nutritional Information

Berries are an excellent source of dietary fibers, potassium, and folates; bananas are rich in proteins and B vitamins. Combine the bountiful benefits of these two ingredients by following this quick and easy DASH brunch recipe:

Ingredients

½ cup granola, plain
1 cup raspberries
2 tablespoons toasted and roughly chopped almonds
2 tablespoons sunflower kernels
2 tablespoons raw honey
2 cups of vanilla fat-free yogurt
2 peaches, small, sliced thinly
4 bananas, halved lengthwise

Preparation

1. Divide the bananas into 4 shallow bowls and top with the rest of the ingredients
2. Serve immediately

Nutritional Information	Per Serving
Sodium	88 milligrams
Calories	340 milligrams
Total Fats	6 grams
Saturated Fats	1 gram
Cholesterol	0 milligram
Carbohydrates	61 grams
Dietary Fibers	9 grams
Proteins	17 grams

Slow Cooker Apple Cinnamon Oatmeal

Preparation 1-hour + slow cooker time (5 hours+++)
Servings 7 (3/4 per cup) servings

Nutritional Information
Apples are rich in dietary fibers and vitamins A and B; cinnamon, on the other hand, is an excellent source for your body's energy! here's how to combine both into a DASH breakfast:

Ingredients
Vegetable oil
1/2 teaspoon cinnamon
1/4 teaspoon iodized salt
1 1/2 cup fat-free milk (the best substitute for almond milk)
1 1/2 cup water
1 1/2 tablespoon butter, sliced into 5-6 pieces
1 tablespoon flax seed, ground
1 cup oats, cooked, steel-cut
2 apples, peeled, cored, sliced into 1/2-inch pieces
2 tablespoons brown sugar

For Garnish
A handful of nuts, roughly chopped
A handful of raisins

Preparation
1. In a slow cooker, coat it with a vegetable oil to cook all the ingredients above (except for the garnishing).

2. Stir and cook while covered on low heat for more than 5 hours (slow cooker time vary).

3. Turn off heat then scoop the oatmeal into the serving bowls.

4. Add the ingredients for garnish.

5. Serve immediately (store leftover oatmeal in the refrigerator).

To Reheat
1. Put a single serving of oatmeal in a microwave-safe bowl.

2. Pour 1/3 cup fat-free milk.

3. Place it in a microwave then heat it for 1 minute.

4. Open oven then stir.

5. Close the oven then continue heating for a few minutes until hot.

Nutritional Information	Per Serving
Sodium	0 milligrams
Calories	149 milligrams
Fats	3.6 grams
Carbohydrates	27.3 grams
Fibers	3.9 grams
Proteins	4.9 grams

Buckwheat Crepes

Preparation 30 minutes   *Servings* 12

Nutritional Information
Make buckwheat crepes in a dash during breakfast by following this quick and easy recipe:

Ingredients
Dairy fat-free milk
3/4 tablespoon flax seed
1 3/4 cup low-fat coconut milk
1/8 teaspoon ground cinnamon
1 dash of stevia
1 pinch of sea salt
1 tablespoon coconut oil
1 cup buckwheat flour, raw *(we highly recommend you to grind your own buckwheat groats)*

For the Filling
A handful of compote
A handful of nut butter
Coconut whipped cream
Granola oats
Baked apple cinnamon

Preparation
1. In a blender, blend buckwheat groat flour, flax seed, coconut milk, sea salt, coconut oil, and stevia.

2. Pulse blender till the consistency thickens; if the texture is watery, add more buckwheat groat flour; if the texture is too thick, add more fat-free dairy milk

3. Coat a non-stick skillet with vegetable oil to cook crepes; to cook, spread to form an even layer.

4. Pour 1/4 cup of batter. Cook until the top bubbles and the edges are fried, flip the other side and cook for a few minutes (repeat this step until all crepes are done).

5. Place cooked buckwheat crepes on a serving platter with a parchment paper or a tissue paper.

6. Serve with your preferred filling

To Restore

1. Store leftover buckwheat crepes in a refrigerator (shelf life can last up to 3 days)

2. To chill, layer crepes between pieces of tissue paper to prevent sticking then leave in the refrigerator.

3. To eat leftover, reheat crepe/s in a 350 °F microwave oven until hot.

Nutritional Information	Per Serving
Sodium	28 milligrams
Calories	71 milligrams
Fibers	1 gram
Fats	3 grams
Proteins	1 gram
Saturated Fats	3 grams
Calcium	0.6%
Iron	2.5%
Potassium	62 milligrams
Carbohydrates	8 grams

Sweet Potato Waffles

Preparation 15 minutes   *Servings* 2

Nutritional Information

Sweet potatoes are a good source of fibers, manganese, calcium, riboflavin, phosphorus and other vitamins and minerals. Here's how to prepare sweet potato waffles for breakfast:

Ingredients

Vegetable oil cooking spray
1/2 cup sweet potato
1/4 teaspoon baking powder
1/4 teaspoon iodized salt
1 tablespoon olive oil
1 tablespoon honey
1 cup rolled oats
1 cup low-fate milk
2 eggs (1 whole egg and 1 egg white only)

Preparation

1. Preheat waffle iron.

2. In a blender, add all ingredients and blend to a puree.

3. Spray preheated waffle iron with vegetable oil cooking spray.

4. Pour 1/3 cup of batter (by batch) on the waffle mold.

5. Cook for 3-4 minutes by batch.

Nutritional Information	Per Serving
Sodium	55 milligrams
Calories	86 milligrams
Cholesterol	0 milligrams
Potassium	337 milligrams
Carbohydrates	20 grams
Dietary fibers	3 grams
Proteins	1.6 grams
Magnesium	6%

DASH French Toast

Preparation 15 minutes   *Servings* 4

Nutritional Information

Did you know that the DASH version of French toast recipe is actually vegetarian and sugar-free?

Ingredients

Pinch of iodized salt
Pinch of cinnamon, powdered
1/2 cup coconut milk, unsweetened
1 packet of stevia
1 teaspoon vanilla extract
2 eggs
2 tablespoon coconut sugar
4 slices of French toast bread

Preparation

1. In a bowl, mix all ingredients together (except for the French toast bread).

2. Spread the mixture evenly on all the French bread toast.

3. In a skillet, heat each side for 5 minutes until light brown.

Nutritional Information	Per Serving
Sodium	0 milligrams
Calories	0 milligrams
Total Fats	11 grams
Saturated Fats	2.7 grams
Polyunsaturated Fats	2.6 grams
Monounsaturated Fats	4.5 grams
Cholesterol	116 milligrams
Sodium	479 milligrams
Potassium	134 milligrams
Total Carbohydrates	25 grams
Proteins	8 grams

Tofu Egg Scramble

Preparation 30 minutes　　　　　*Servings* 2
Nutritional Information
Tofu is an excellent source of proteins and contains nine types of amino acids; eating an egg is also a great source of proteins. Combine the two ingredients to create a DASH breakfast recipe:

Ingredients for Egg Scramble
1/2 red pepper, sliced thinly
1/4 thinly-sliced red onion
2 cups of kale, roughly chopped
2 tablespoons olive oil
8 ounces tofu, extra firm

Ingredients for Sauce
Water, as needed
1/2 teaspoon sea salt
1/2 teaspoon garlic powder
1/2 teaspoon cumin powder
1/4 teaspoon chili powder
1/4 teaspoon turmeric
Ingredients for Garnish
Salsa
Cilantro
Hot sauce
Potatoes, baked

Preparation
1. Pat dry tofu and roll on a clean and absorbent towel; press it in a cast-iron skillet for 15 minutes.

2. in a bowl, prepare the sauce by mixing all the ingredients together; set aside.

3. In a skillet, heat olive oil over medium heat to sauté onion and red pepper; once tender, add all the vegetables then

put a dash of salt and pepper. Stir frequently while cooking until tender for 5 minutes.

4. Add the kale and cover to steam for a few minutes.

5. unwrap the tofu then use a fork to crumble into small pieces.

6. Using a spatula, set the vegetables to one side of the pan then add tofu; sauté for a few minutes.

7. Pour a generous amount of sauce on the tofu and drizzle some on the vegetables. Stir to distribute the sauce evenly; cook for 5 more minutes until tofu is light brown.

8. Serve together with your preferred garnish.

To Reheat
1. Store tofu scramble in a freezer (shelf life can last up to a month).

2. Reheat on a stovetop or microwave oven and serve hot.

Nutritional Information	Per Serving
Sodium	516 milligrams
Calories	252 milligrams
Fats	19 grams
Sugar	2.5 grams
Proteins	12 grams
Carbohydrates	12.7 grams
Dietary Fiber	3 grams

Bella Mushroom and Spinach Omelet

Preparation 20 minutes   *Servings* 1
Nutritional Information
The Bella mushroom is a great source of proteins and dietary fibers; spinach is also a good source of proteins and carbohydrates; an egg is also an excellent source of proteins. this protein-packed DASH breakfast can be done quickly and easily:

Ingredients
Vegetable oil cooking spray
1/4 cup thinly sliced red onion
1 1/2 cup spinach
1 egg, large
1 ounce goat cheese
1 tablespoon olive oil
1 diced green onion for garnish
2 egg whites
5 thinly sliced baby Bella mushrooms

Preparation
1. Heat a skillet to medium, then spray the vegetable oil to sauté red onions until translucent.

2. Add the mushrooms and sauté until light brown.

3. Add the spinach, season with salt and pepper, then sauté until wilted.

4. Heat another skillet and spray with a vegetable oil cooking spray.

5. Put the eggs in a bowl and whisk.

6. Pour the egg mixture into the skillet; place mushroom-spinach mixture on one side of the egg and cover with the other side of the egg to form an omelet.

7. Cook for a few minutes and transfer to a serving platter.

8. Sprinkle green onions for garnish and serve

Nutritional Information	Per Serving
Sodium	332 milligrams
Calories	412 milligrams
Sugar	8 grams
Fats	29 grams
Carbohydrates	18 grams
Dietary Fibers	4 grams
Proteins	25 grams
Cholesterol	199 grams

Chapter 4 – A Dash of Enticing Appetizers

With these DASH recipes, you can cook and eat the most enticing appetizers without the stress of ruining your healthy appetite.

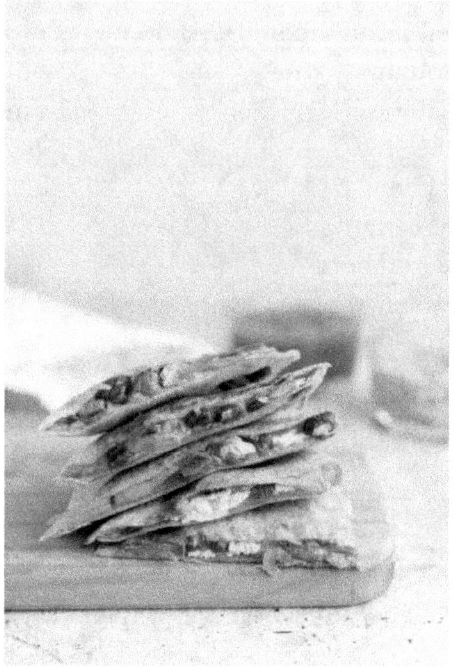

Chicken Quesadillas

Preparation 30 minutes   *Servings* 6

Nutritional Information

Chicken is rich in meat proteins, combined with vegetables for a DASH diet. Chicken Quesadillas are a flavorful and finger-licking appetizer that is also a great party food.

Ingredients

½ cup salsa
1 cup tomatoes, minced
1 cup cilantro, minced
1 cup onions, minced
4 ounces boneless, skinless chicken breasts

6 pieces of whole wheat 8-inch tortillas

Preparation
1. Chop each chicken breast to bite-sized.
2. Place chicken and onions in a non-stick frying pan, then sauté until thoroughly cooked and tender.
3. Remove from heat; stir in tomatoes, cilantro, and salsa.
4. To assemble, use a serving platter. Rub one part of the tortilla with water then lay it flat and spread ½ cup of chicken mixture; leave ½ inch free around the rim; sprinkle with shredded cheese and fold the tortilla in half.
5. Transfer the chicken quesadillas onto a baking pan lined with a parchment paper.
6. Lightly coat with vegetable oil and bake for up to ten minutes or until the quesadillas turn light brown.
7. Slice in half or serve immediately as is.

Nutritional Information	Per Serving
Calories	298 milligrams
Cholesterol	70 milligrams
Sodium	524 milligrams
Carbohydrates	25 grams
Saturated Fats	5 grams
Proteins	27 grams

Italian Sausage Zucchini Boats

Preparation 1-hour   *Servings* 6
Nutritional Information
Zucchini is a great source of potassium and dietary fibers, while sausages are rich in proteins.

Ingredients
Vegetable oil
1/3 cup Parmesan grated cheese
1/3 cup minced parsley
1/4 teaspoon ground black pepper
3/4 cup part-skim shredded mozzarella cheese
1 pound Italian sausage, casing removed
1 cup Panko breadcrumbs
2 tablespoons oregano, minced
2 tablespoons basil, minced
2 medium, cored, sliced tomatoes
6 medium zucchini

Preparation
1. Preheat oven to 360 °F.

2. Chop zucchini in half lengthwise, then scoop out the pulp, leaving only 1/4 to form a boat.

3. Place the zucchini boats in a microwave-safe oven (per batch depending on the microwave's capacity); turn on to medium heat and microwave covered for 3 minutes until crisp.

4. In a skillet, heat vegetable oil to cook zucchini pulp and sausage for 5-10 minutes until the sausage is brownish ; break the sausage to bite-sized.

5. Add tomatoes, Panko breadcrumbs, Parmesan cheese, pepper, and other herbs.

6. Spoon the filling onto the zucchini boats.

7. Transfer the zucchini boats onto a baking pan and place it in a microwave oven.

8. Bake covered for 15-20 minutes until the zucchini boats are tender.

9. Open the oven to sprinkle mozzarella cheese, then bake uncovered for 5-10 minutes until the cheese melts.

10. Remove from the oven and sprinkle with minced parsley for garnish.

11. Serve on a platter.

Nutritional Information	Per Serving
Sodium	485 milligrams
Calories	206 milligrams
Fats	9 grams
Cholesterol	39 milligrams
Carbohydrates	16 grams
Saturated Fats	3 grams
Sugar	5 grams
Dietary Fibers	3 grams
Proteins	17 grams

Cherry-Chicken Lettuce Cups

Preparation 30 minutes   *Servings* 4
Nutritional Information
Cherries aids in digestion, control blood sugar, and promote
weight loss. Chicken is a good source of proteins; lettuce is rich in
minerals. Combine the three ingredients to create an enticing
DASH appetizer by following the recipe below:

Ingredients
Vegetable oil cooking spray
3/4 pound boneless, skinless, cubed chicken breast
1/3 cup coarsely chopped almonds
1/4 teaspoon iodized salt
1/4 teaspoon ground black pepper
1 teaspoon ground ginger
1 1/2 cup carrots, shredded
1 1/4 cup sweet cherries, pitted, coarsely chopped
1 tablespoon raw honey
2 teaspoon olive oil
2 tablespoons rice vinegar
2 tablespoons low sodium teriyaki sauce
4 green onions, minced
8 small lettuce leaf pieces
Preparation
1. Season chicken with salt and pepper

2. Coat a non-stick skillet with vegetable oil cooking spray
    and heat over medium heat.

3. Cook chicken cubes until light brown.

4. Remove chicken from heat then stir in carrots, cherries,
    green onions, and almonds.

5. In another bowl, mix teriyaki sauce, vinegar, and honey
    together; pour onto the chicken cubes to coat.

6. Divide seasoned chicken cubes among the lettuce leaves, then fold over to form a cup.

7. Serve immediately on a platter.

Nutritional Information	Per Serving
Sodium	381 milligrams
Calories	257 milligrams
Fats	10 grams
Saturated Fats	1 gram
Cholesterol	47 milligrams
Carbohydrates	22 grams
Sugar	15 grams
Dietary Fibers	4 grams
Proteins	21 grams

Turkey Barbecue Burger

Preparation 30 minutes   *Servings* 4
Nutritional Information
With the DASH Diet, combining a barbecue and burger is totally possible and 100% healthy! Add turkey, which is rich in tryptophan content that boosts healthy serotonin levels. Tryptophan promotes alertness and a good mood throughout the day, so have a bite by following the recipe below:

Ingredients
1/4 cup chopped basil
1/4 teaspoon garlic salt
1/8 teaspoon ground black pepper
1 pound lean ground turkey
1 clove of minced garlic
1 thinly sliced tomato
1 slice provolone cheese
1 small thinly sliced red onion
2 tablespoons oat bran
3 tablespoons smoke-flavored mesquite barbecue sauce
4 split whole wheat hamburger buns
Preparation
1. Combine barbecue sauce, oat bran, garlic, garlic salt, pepper, and basil in a bowl.

2. Add ground turkey and form 1/2-inch thick burger patties.

3. Lightly grease a grill rack with vegetable oil and grill for 5-10 minutes on each side; grill hamburger buns till toasted.

4. Sandwich the turkey patty with your preferred toppings.

5. Serve on a platter.

Nutritional Information	Per Serving
Sodium	381 milligrams
Calories	257 milligrams
Fats	10 grams
Saturated Fats	1 gram
Cholesterol	47 milligrams
Carbohydrates	22 grams
Sugar	15 grams
Dietary Fibers	4 grams
Proteins	21 grams

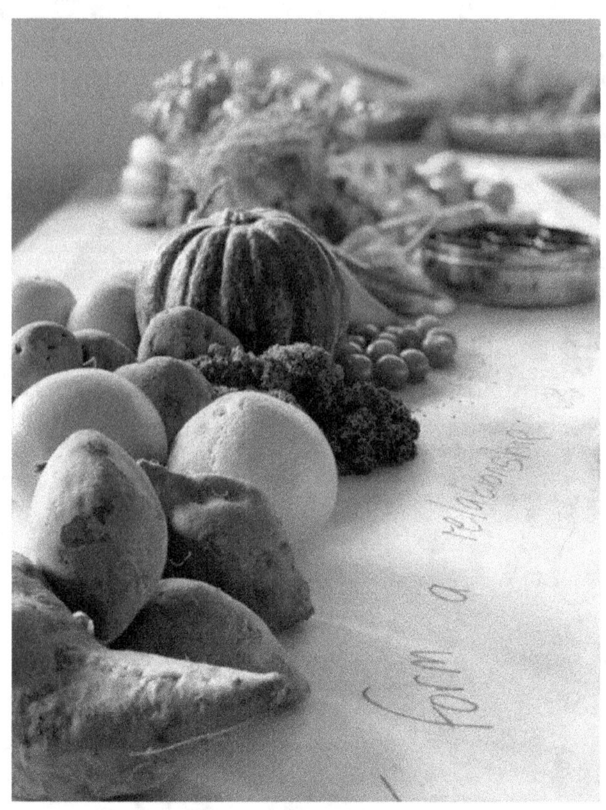

Sweet Potato and Chickpea Pita Doner

Preparation 30 minutes   *Servings* 6

Nutritional Information

Sweet potatoes contain high amounts of dietary fibers and potassium; chickpeas, on the other hand, are rich in proteins. Sandwich the two ingredients in a pita doner with this enticing DASH appetizer recipe below:

Ingredients

1/2 teaspoon iodized salt

¼ cup cilantro, minced

1 medium red onion sliced in strips

1 cup plain Greek yogurt

1 tablespoon lemon juice extract

1 teaspoon ground cumin

2 cups baby spinach

2 minced garlic cloves

2 peeled, cubed pieces of sweet potatoes, medium (about 1 ¼ pound)

2 cans (15 ounces each) chickpeas, rinsed and drained

2 teaspoons garam masala

3 tablespoons canola oil

12 pieces of halved, warmed whole wheat pita pocket

Preparation

1. Preheat oven to 400 °F.
2. Place the sweet potatoes in a microwave-safe bowl and put it in a microwave oven; turn the heat on high and microwave for 5 minutes.
3. Open the oven, then add the chickpeas and onion; drizzle the canola oil, garam masala, and ¼ teaspoon iodized salt.
4. Transfer contents to a baking pan lined with parchment paper; roast for 15 minutes until the sweet potatoes are tender.
5. Once done roasting, set aside and allow to cool.
6. Put garlic and the remaining canola oil in a microwave-safe bowl; place it in the microwave oven and turn to high heat for a minute or two until the garlic is light brown.
7. Drizzle the Greek yogurt, cumin, lemon juice extract, and remaining iodized salt.
8. Toss sweet potatoes with baby spinach.
9. Scoop it into the pita breads, drizzle with sauce and top with cilantro.
10. Serve with a tissue paper as the packaging.

Nutritional Information	Per Serving
Sodium	662 milligrams
Calories	462 milligrams
Fats	15 grams
Saturated Fats	3 grams
Cholesterol	10 milligrams
Carbohydrates	72 grams
Sugar	13 grams
Dietary Fibers	12 grams
Proteins	14 grams

Sesame Chicken Veggie Tortilla Wraps

Preparation 30 minutes   *Servings* 8

Nutritional Information

Sesame chicken is a good source of proteins and dietary fibers; wrap it with vegetables for a nutritiously good DASH appetizer.

Main Ingredient

1 cup shelled, frozen edamame

Dressing Ingredients

½ teaspoon ground ginger

¼ teaspoon iodized salt

1/8 teaspoon ground black pepper

1 teaspoon sesame oil

2 tablespoons orange juice extract

2 tablespoons olive oil

Ingredients for the Wraps

½ cup carrots, shredded

½ cup sweet red pepper, sliced thinly

1 cup chicken breast, cooked, chopped to bite-sized bits

1 cup cucumber, thinly sliced

1 cup sugar snap peas, chopped

2 cups baby spinach

8 whole wheat, room temperature tortilla pieces (8-inches in size),

Preparation

1. Cook the edamame according to the packaging instructions; drain, wash with cold water then drain completely.
2. Whisk edamame in a bowl with the dressing ingredients.
3. Toss the seasoned edamame with the chicken in a separate bowl.
4. Put ½ cup of mixture on each tortilla wrap.
5. Fold the tortilla on the bottom and on the edges to wrap and roll up the mixture.
6. Serve on a platter.

Nutritional Information	Per Serving
Sodium	229 milligrams
Calories	214 milligrams
Fats	7 grams
Saturated Fats	1 gram
Cholesterol	13 milligrams
Carbohydrates	28 grams
Sugar	2 grams
Dietary Fibers	5 grams
Proteins	12 grams

Lime Chicken Tacos

Preparation 5 hours and 30 minutes   *Servings* 12

Nutritional Information
Lime chicken tacos are not only appetizing but are perfect for weight watchers. They are packed with proteins, which promotes weight loss, improves the digestive system, lowers blood sugar levels, reduces the risk of heart disease, and much more!

Ingredients
A handful of jalapeños
Cheese
1 cup shredded lettuce
1 lime zest
1 tablespoon powdered chili
1 cup thawed frozen corn
1 cup salsa
1 cup sour cream
1 ½ pound skinless, boneless, halved chicken breast
3 tablespoons lime juice extract
12 pieces of warmed fat-free flour tortilla wraps

Preparation
1. Place chicken, lime juice and chili powder in a 3-quart slow cooker.
2. Cook covered on low heat for about 5 hours until the chicken is tender.
3. Remove chicken from the slow cooker, set aside and allow to cool; once the chicken is warm, shred meat using a stainless-steel fork, then put it back in the slow cooker.
4. Add the corn and salsa; cook covered on low heat for 30 minutes.
5. Place the filling on the tortillas, then add the condiments: sour cream, lettuce, jalapeños, and cheese.

Nutritional Information	Per Serving
Sodium	674 milligrams
Calories	291 milligrams
Fats	3 grams
Saturated Fats	1 gram
Cholesterol	63 milligrams
Carbohydrates	37 grams
Sugar	2 grams
Dietary Fibers	2 grams
Proteins	28 grams

Black Bean Burger

Preparation 45 minutes   *Servings* 6
Nutritional Information
Black beans are a great source of molybdenum, a type of nutritious minerals. Black beans also contain iron, magnesium, manganese, phosphorus, vitamin B1, and much more! Add a DASH of black in your life with a black bean burger by following the recipe below:

Ingredients
Vegetable oil
Tomato ketchup
Dash of ground black pepper
½ medium coarsely chopped yellow onion
½ teaspoon red pepper flakes
½ cup breadcrumbs
½ cup grated cheese
1 cup shredded lettuce
1 thinly sliced tomato
1 tablespoon minced garlic
1 tablespoon Sriracha
1 egg
2 (15 ounces each) cans of black beans, rinsed, drained, equally divided
2 teaspoons coarsely chopped parsley leaves
6 pieces of whole grain burger buns,
Preparation
1. Preheat a grill pan on medium heat and coat it with vegetable oil.
2. Pulse yellow onion and garlic in a blender, followed by the black beans, egg, cilantro, parsley, and red pepper flakes; pulse to make a filling. Transfer contents to a bowl.
3. Add the remaining black beans from the can and the breadcrumbs; season with pepper and mix to coat the beans.

4. Reserve 1/3cup of the coated black beans; divide the remaining black bean mixture equally to form a burger patty.
5. Place black bean patties on the grill over medium heat and cook 5 minutes on each side; toast the hamburger buns on the grill.
6. Put the black bean burger patty on the bun; top it with lettuce, tomatoes, and tomato ketchup.
7. Serve on a platter.

Nutritional Information	Per Serving
Sodium	9 milligrams
Calories	339 milligrams
Saturated Fats	0.2 grams
Polyunsaturated Fats	0.4 grams
Monounsaturated Fats	0.1grams
Cholesterol	0 milligrams
Potassium	1,500 milligrams
Total Carbohydrates	63 grams
Dietary Fibers	16 grams
Sugar	2.1 grams
Proteins	21 grams

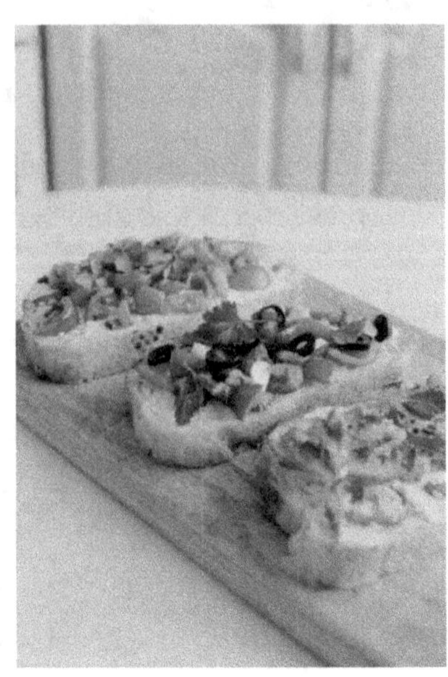

Tomato and Basil Bruschetta

Preparation 30 minutes   *Servings* 6

Nutritional Information

Tomatoes are rich in dietary fibers and carbohydrates, while basil is rich in vitamins A, C, K, calcium, iron, potassium, and magnesium.

Ingredients

½ piece whole grain baguette, sliced into 6 ½-inch thick diagonal slices

½ cup diced fennel

1 teaspoon olive oil

1 tablespoon coarsely chopped parsley

1 teaspoon black pepper

2 teaspoons balsamic vinegar

2 tablespoons basil, coarsely chopped

2 minced garlic cloves

3 pieces of tomato, diced

Preparation

1. Preheat oven to 400 °F
2. Toast baguettes until it turns light brown .
3. Mix all remaining ingredients in a bowl.
4. Scoop the mixture evenly over each toasted baguette.
5. Serve on a platter immediately.

Nutritional Information	Per Serving
Sodium	123 milligrams
Calories	110 milligrams
Total Fats	2 grams
Carbohydrates	20 grams
Proteins	3 grams
Dietary Fibers	4 grams

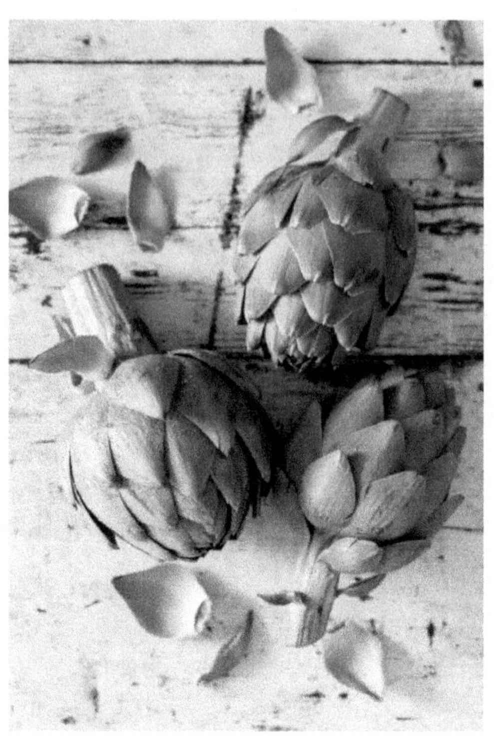

Artichoke Hearts Spinach Dip

Preparation 1-hour   *Servings* N/A
Nutritional Information
Artichoke hearts are rich in fibers, folates, magnesium, potassium, and Vitamin C. Spinach contains macronutrients such as proteins, fibers, carbohydrates and much more! You are going to love this DASH appetizer full of heart; just follow the recipe below:

Ingredients
½ cup low fat sour cream
1 tablespoon black pepper
1 teaspoon thyme, minced
1 tablespoon minced parsley
1 cup white beans, rinsed
2 tablespoons Parmesan cheese
2 minced garlic cloves

2 cups artichoke hearts

4 cups coarsely chopped spinach

Preparation

1. Mix all the ingredients in a bowl.
2. Transfer the mixture into a ceramic dish.
3. Bake it in the oven at 350 °F for 30 minutes.
4. Serve the artichoke hearts spinach dip with a whole grain bread or plain white crackers.

Nutritional Information	Per Serving
Sodium	71 milligrams
Calories	94 milligrams
Total Fats	2 grams
Carbohydrates	14 grams
Dietary Fibers	6 grams
Proteins	5 grams
Sugar	0 milligrams

Chicken Enchiladas

Preparation 4 hours and 10 minutes   *Servings* 4
Nutritional Information
Chicken is rich in proteins, and everybody loves it prepared in enchiladas. Here's how:

Ingredients
½ cup low sodium salsa
½ cup Mexican style cheese
½ teaspoon ground cumin
1 pound skinless, boneless, halved chicken breast
1 can (10 ounces) of low-fat, low-sodium cream of chicken soup
1 teaspoon powdered chili,
4 cups of baby lettuce
8 pieces of (6-inch) corn tortillas, warmed

Preparation
1. Place the chicken breasts in a 1 ½ quart slow cooker,.
2. Mix the cream of chicken soup, salsa, cumin, and chili powder in a bowl.
3. Drizzle the chicken soup mixture over the chicken in the slow cooker; cook covered for up to 4 hours.
4. Remove chicken from the slow cooker and transfer to a bowl.
5. Shred the chicken meat with a stainless-steel fork; drizzle half the chicken sauce from the slow cooker onto the shredded chicken, toss to coat.
6. Line a serving platter with lettuce and place about ½ cup the chicken mixture and 1 teaspoon shredded cheese on the middle of each tortilla and roll it up to wrap.
7. Spoon the remaining chicken sauce and cheese over the enchiladas and serve immediately.

To Reheat

1. To reheat the chicken enchiladas, preheat oven to 350 °F.
2. Wrap the tortillas tightly in aluminum foil.
3. Put it in the oven and bake for 10 minutes.

Nutritional Information	Per Serving
Sodium	599 milligrams
Calories	271 milligrams
Fats	9 grams
Saturated Fats	4 grams
Dietary Fibers	3 grams
Carbohydrates	24 grams
Proteins	22 grams
Folic Acid (mcg folate)	17 micrograms
Cholesterol	63 milligrams
Sugar	6 grams
Calcium	129 milligrams
Iron	1 milligram
Potassium	810 milligrams

DASH Acorn Squash Rings

Preparation 1-hour *Servings*
Nutritional Information
Squash serve as immunity boosters and promote blood circulation and a healthy heart. They are an excellent source of numerous nutrients such as proteins, calcium, folates, fibers, potassium, magnesium, and much more!
Here's how to make DASH delicate squash rings:

Ingredients
¼ teaspoon iodized salt
1/8 teaspoon ground black pepper
¾ cup low sodium vegetable broth
1 teaspoon rosemary, snipped
2 tablespoons light stick butter
2 thinly sliced garlic cloves
2 (about 2 pounds) medium acorn squash

Preparation
1. Preheat oven to 350 °F.
2. Slice the squash in half lengthwise; remove and discard the seeds.
3. Transfer the halved squash with the cut sides down onto a cutting board; cut to 1-inch crosswise slices. Repeat the same step for all the squash.
4. Pour the vegetable broth into a 2-quart rectangular baking dish; overlap the squash and garlic slices; dash with salt and pepper.
5. Put it in a microwave oven then bake covered for about 40 minutes; bake uncovered until the squash rings are tender for 10-15 minutes.
6. Transfer the squash rings to a serving platter and reserve the liquid in the baking dish.

7. Mix butter and rosemary snips with the liquid in the baking
    dish, scoop it over the squash rings on the platter and
    serve immediately.

Nutritional Information	Per Serving
Sodium	205 milligrams
Calories	155 milligrams
Fats	3 grams
Saturated Fats	2 grams
Dietary Fibers	3 grams
Carbohydrates	25 grams
Proteins	2 grams
Folates	39 micrograms
Cholesterol	8 milligrams
Sugar	0 milligrams
Calcium	82 milligrams
Iron	2 milligrams
Potassium	826 milligrams

DASH Delicata Squash Rounds

Preparation 40 minutes　　　　　　*Servings N/A*
Nutritional Information

Apart from treating hypertension, Delicata Squash Rounds are the perfect DASH-ing appetizer for weight watchers. Here's how to make "delicate" DASH squash rounds:

Ingredients
½ tablespoon iodized salt
¼ cup sour cream
¾ cup Plain Greek yogurt
1 tablespoon lemon juice
1 Delicata squash, medium, sliced into ½-inch thick rings
1 teaspoon cumin, powdered
1 teaspoon paprika
1 tablespoon minced garlic
2 tablespoon minced dill
2 tablespoons olive oil

Dipping Ingredients
Broccoli florets
Baby carrots
Bell pepper
Cucumber
Other favorite vegetables

Preparation
1. Preheat oven to 375 °F.
2. In a bowl, mix Greek yogurt, lemon juice extract, dill, sour cream, and iodized salt; set aside.
3. In another bowl, combine paprika, remaining garlic, salt, and olive oil; set aside.
4. Chop and core the Delicata squash and slice to ½-inch thick rings; lay them on a bowl and coat with garlic olive oil.

5. Spread the Delicata squash rings in a baking pan and place in a microwave oven; bake until tender and crisp for about 20-25 minutes.

6. Remove from the oven and serve with the dip and your preferred vegetables.

Nutritional Information	Per Serving
Sodium	8 milligrams
Calories	17 milligrams
Total Fats	0.3 grams
Saturated Fats	0.1 gram
Monounsaturated fats	0 grams
Trans Fats	0 grams
Cholesterol	0 milligrams
Potassium	261 milligrams
Total Carbohydrates	3.1 grams
Dietary Fibers	1 gram
Sugar	2.5 grams
Proteins	1.2 grams

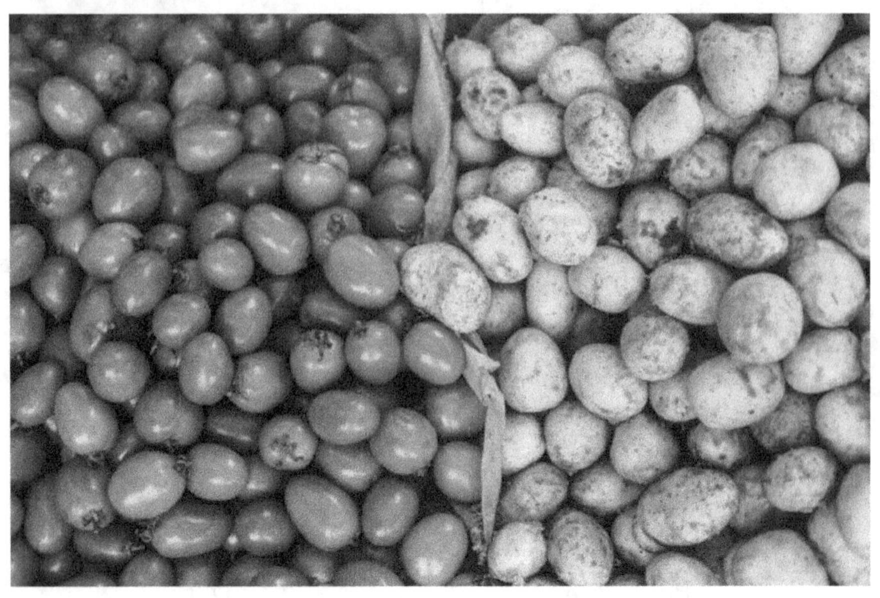

Cottage Cheese and Roasted Tomato Topped Potatoes

Preparation 25 minutes   *Servings* 1
Nutritional Information
Tomatoes are rich in four major carotenoids: alpha, beta-carotene, lutein, and lycopene; potatoes, on the other hand are rich in phytonutrients that have antioxidant activities. Combine the two ingredients with this appetizing DASH recipe below:

Ingredients
½ cup red cherry tomatoes
½ cup yellow cherry tomatoes
¼ cup cottage cheese, low-fat
1 teaspoon chives, snipped
1 piece (6 pounds) of russet potato, baked
2 teaspoons olive oil

Preparation
1. Preheat oven to 425 °F

2. In a 2-quart baking dish, coat the cherry tomatoes with olive oil
3. Put it in a microwave oven and roast until the cherry tomatoes crack open for 30 minutes.
4. Top the russet potato with cottage cheese, roasted tomatoes, and chives
5. Serve immediately on a platter

Nutritional Information	Per Serving
Sodium	208 milligrams
Calories	304 milligrams
Fats	11 grams
Saturated Fats	2 grams
Dietary Fibers	5 grams
Carbohydrates	42 grams
Proteins	11 grams
Folates	67 micrograms
Cholesterol	7 milligrams
Sugar	5 grams
Added Sugar	9 grams
Vitamin C	24 milligrams
Calcium	103 milligrams
Iron	2 milligrams
Potassium	1,205 milligrams

Cheesy Broccoli Baked Potato Hams

Preparation 10 minutes   *Servings* 1
Nutritional Information
Broccoli is a great source of beta-carotene and B vitamins. Potatoes are rich in phytonutrients; balance this enticing DASH appetizer with ham that is rich in proteins and fibers to give you a fulfilling dish.

Ingredients
½ cup small broccoli florets
¼ cup shredded, low-fat cheddar cheese
1 cup low sodium cubed ham
1 tablespoon non-fat Plain Greek yogurt
1 (6 ounces) baked russet potato

Preparation
1. Put all the ingredients in a microwave-safe bowl.
2. Place it in a microwave oven at a medium heat and cook it until tender.
3. Remove from the microwave oven and serve on a platter.

Nutritional Information	Per Serving
Sodium	464 milligrams
Calories	298 milligrams
Fats	7 grams
Saturated Fats	4 grams
Dietary Fibers	5 grams
Carbohydrates	41 grams
Proteins	19 grams
Folates	74 micrograms
Cholesterol	32 milligrams
Sugar	4 grams
Added Sugar	0 grams
Vitamin C	55 grams
Calcium	475 milligrams
Iron	2 milligrams
Potassium	1,079 milligrams

Chapter 5 – A Dash of Mouthwatering Main Courses

Eat the most mouthwatering main courses without feeling any pressure to eat unhealthily. Here are the DASH diet versions of your everyday favorite main courses.

Baked Chicken with Onion, Tarragon, and Wild Rice

Preparation 2 hours *Servings* 6
Nutritional Information
This DASH baked chicken recipe is moist and flavorful as a result of a slow cooking method; the delicate taste of tarragon and other nutritious ingredients complements the dish perfectly.

Ingredients
¾ cup uncooked long grain rice
¾ cup uncooked wild rice
1 pound boneless, skinless, halved chicken breasts
1 ½ cup minced celery
1 ½ cup whole pearl onions
1 ½ cup dry white wine
1 teaspoon tarragon
2 cups unsalted chicken broth

Preparation
1. Preheat oven to 300 °F.
2. In a non-stick frying pan, combine chicken broth, chicken, tarragon, celery, and onion. Cook on medium heat until the contents are tender and cooked thoroughly for about ten minutes; set aside and allow to cool.
3. In a baking dish, combine wine, remaining chicken broth, and wild rice; soak for 30 minutes.
4. Place cooked chicken and vegetables in a baking pan lined with parchment paper, cover with aluminum foil and bake for at least an hour.

5. Check frequently and pour in more broth if the rice is too dry.
6. Serve immediately.

Nutritional Information	Per Serving
Carbohydrates	37 grams
Dietary Fibers	2 grams
Sodium	180 milligrams
Saturated Fats	1 grams
Total Fats	3 grams
Cholesterol	53 milligrams
Proteins	21 milligrams
Monounsaturated Fats	1 grams
Calories	330

Beefy Veggie Soup

Preparation 1 hour   *Servings* 8
Nutritional Information
This beefy veggie DASH soup contains all the ingredients that will definitely help you treat your high blood pressure and give you the energy you need for the entire day. Here's how to cook this beefy soup full of veggies:

Ingredients
Parmesan grated cheese (optional)
½ cup frozen cut green beans
½ teaspoon dried oregano
¼ teaspoon iodized salt
¼ teaspoon ground black pepper
¼ cup tomato paste
1 ½ cup shredded cabbage
1 can (14 ½ pounds) of diced tomatoes
1 (1/2 pound) 90% lean ground beef
1 teaspoon dried basil
1 medium coarsely chopped zucchini
1 medium onion, sliced into rings
1 medium (about 5 ounces) cubed red potato
2 minced garlic cloves
2 ribs of minced celery
4 cans (14 ½ ounces) low sodium beef broth
5 julienned carrot pieces

Preparation
1. In a 6-quart stockpot, cook beef, garlic and onion over medium heat for 5-8 minutes until the beef is no longer pinkish; break the beef into bite-sized pieces and drain the liquids.
2. Add the celery and carrots, cook and stir frequently until tender for 5-8 minutes
3. Stir in the tomato paste and cook for a minute longer.

4. Add the tomatoes, potatoes, zucchini, cabbage, green beans, beef broth, and seasoning; bring to a boil.
5. Once the soup bubbles, reduce the heat and simmer covered until the vegetables are tender for about 30-40 minutes.
6. Serve and top with Parmesan cheese if desired.

Nutritional Information	Per Serving
Sodium	621 milligrams
Calories	207 milligrams
Fats	7 grams
Saturated Fats	3 grams
Cholesterol	57 milligrams
Carbohydrates	14 grams
Sugar	7 grams
Dietary Fibers	3 grams
Proteins	21 grams

Strawberry Blue Cheese Steak

Preparation 30 minutes   *Servings* 4
Nutritional Information
Feeling "blue" because of your hypertension? Try a "berry" different kind of steak! Follow the recipe below for the DASH version of steak:

Ingredients
Vegetable oil
Low-fat balsamic vinaigrette,
½ teaspoon iodized salt
¼ teaspoon ground black pepper
¼ cup thinly sliced red onion
¼ cup crumbled blue cheese
¼ cup toasted walnuts
1 bunch of romaine lettuce, torn
1 slab (about ¾ inch thick and 1 pound) beef top sirloin steak
2 teaspoon olive oil
2 cups of strawberries, halved
2 tablespoons lime juice extract

Preparation
1. Season steak with salt and pepper.
2. Coat a skillet with vegetable oil and cook steak over medium heat until it reaches your desired doneness (for medium-rare, a thermometer should reach 135 degrees, for medium 140 degrees, and for medium-well 145 degrees).
3. Remove steak from the skillet and allow to sit for 5 minutes; slice the beef steak to bite-size strips and coat with lime juice extract.
4. On a serving platter, combine romaine lettuce, strawberries, onions, and top it with steak; sprinkle with blue cheese and walnuts.
5. Serve with balsamic vinaigrette.

Nutritional Information	Per Serving
Sodium	452 milligrams
Calories	289 milligrams
Fats	15 grams
Saturated Fats	4 grams
Cholesterol	52 milligrams
Carbohydrates	12 grams
Sugar	5 grams
Dietary Fibers	4 grams
Proteins	29 grams

Poached Salmon Miso

Preparation 1-hour   *Servings* 4
Nutritional Information
Salmon is an excellent source of omega-3 fatty acids, antioxidant amino acid, taurine, choline, biotin, pantothenic acid, and much more! Here's how to cook poached salmon miso the DASH way:

Ingredients
¾ cup farro
¼ teaspoon ground black pepper
1 ¼ pound wild Alaskan salmon fillet, skinned, sliced into 1-inch pieces
1 tablespoon extra-virgin coconut oil
1 bunch of asparagus, trimmed and chopped to 1-inch pieces
2 minced garlic cloves
2 cups low sodium chicken broth
2 cups of leeks, white and light green parts only, halved, sliced thinly
3 cups of water
3 tablespoons thinly sliced basil
3 tablespoons sweet, mild flavored white miso

Preparation
1. In a saucepan, combine farro and water and bring to a boil over high heat; once it bubbles, reduce to simmer while covered, cook until tender and juicy for about 30 minutes drain completely, and set aside.
2. Fifteen minutes after starting the farro water, warm the extra-virgin coconut oil over medium heat in the saucepan.
3. Add the leeks and cook for 2 minutes, stirring to soften.
4. Add the garlic and asparagus; cook, stirring until the asparagus turn light green
5. Add the white miso and chicken broth, turn the heat to high and bring to a boil

6. Reduce the heat to medium and stir in salmon; simmer for
    3 minutes
7. Remove from heat, then mix the ground black pepper and
    basil
8. Divide the poached salmon miso into 4 shallow bowls and
    serve immediately

Nutritional Information	Per Serving
Sodium	432 milligrams
Calories	407 milligrams
Fats	11 grams
Saturated Fats	2 grams
Dietary Fibers	5 grams
Carbohydrates	40 grams
Proteins	37 grams
Folates	129 micrograms
Cholesterol	66 milligrams
Sugar	4 grams
Added Sugar	0 grams
Calcium	125 milligrams
Iron	3 milligrams
Potassium	847 milligrams

Seared Chicken with Mango Salsa

Preparation 1-hour   *Servings* 4
Nutritional Information
Chicken is a good source of proteins, enhanced by the tangy flavor of mango, which is rich in multivitamins, potassium, and folates. Here it is paired with a different kind of spaghetti made of squash, a good source of omega-3 fatty acids, pantothenic acid, and much more! Here's how to make this unique DASH party lunch:

Ingredients
½ cup diced red onion
¼ cup chopped cilantro
¼ cup almonds, chopped, toasted
1 ¼ teaspoon kosher salt
1 spaghetti squash (3 pounds), halved lengthwise, seeds removed
1 ripe peeled, diced mango
1 minced jalapeño, seeds removed
1 tablespoon brown sugar
2 (8 ounces) boneless, skinless, trimmed, halved chicken breasts
2 tablespoons canola oil
2 tablespoons red wine vinegar
2 tablespoons water

Preparation
1. In a bowl, mix mango, onion, cilantro, jalapeño, vinegar, brown sugar, and salt; set aside.
2. Place the squash with its cut-side down in a microwave-safe dish, add water.
3. Microwave uncovered on high until the squash is tender for 10-15 minutes.
4. Using a meat mallet, pound the chicken on its smooth side, then season with salt.

5. Heat canola oil at medium-high temperature in a skillet; cook the chicken for 5 minutes on each side.

6. Once the squash is cooked, use a stainless fork to scrape off and form spaghetti strips; put the spaghetti squash into a bowl.

7. Toss with the remaining canola oil and salt.

8. Serve the spaghetti squash with the chicken and mango salsa; top with almonds.

Nutritional Information	Per Serving
Sodium	461 milligrams
Calories	366 milligrams
Fats	13 grams
Saturated Fats	7 grams
Dietary Fibers	7 grams
Carbohydrates	38 grams
Proteins	27 grams
Folates	70 micrograms
Cholesterol	63 milligrams
Sugar	23 grams
Added sugar	3 grams
Calcium	106 milligrams
Iron	2 milligrams
Potassium	761 milligrams

Barbecue Pork Chops with Roasted Spinach and Kale

Preparation 1-hour   *Servings* 4
Nutritional Information
Love barbecue? Then DASH some barbecue flavor in a heart-healthy lunch by adding spinach and kale. Pork is rich in proteins. Spinach contains macro-nutrients, while kale contains fibers and other nutrients.

Ingredients
½ teaspoon iodized salt
¼ teaspoon garlic powder
1 ½ pound red potatoes, sliced into 1-inch pieces
1 ½ pound yellow potatoes, sliced into 1-inch pieces
1 teaspoon powdered chili
1 teaspoon paprika
2 (8-10 pounds) boneless, trimmed pork chops
2 tablespoons canola oil
2 tablespoons water
4 tablespoons barbecue sauce
4 cups of kale, stems trimmed, chopped

Preparation
1. Preheat oven to 425 °F.
2. Lay 2 (24-inch long) sheets of aluminum foil on your prepping surface, overlap one about halfway over the other to make a long and wide sheet; lightly coat with canola oil.
3. Toss the potatoes and kale in a bowl using a tablespoon greased with the canola oil, paprika, garlic powder, chili powder, and salt.
4. Mound the vegetables on the center of the aluminum foil.
5. Wrap up the aluminum foil to form a packet and place it on a baking sheet.
6. Put it in the preheated oven, then roast the potatoes until tender for about 25 minutes.

7. Heat the remaining tablespoon of oil in a skillet over medium-high heat; sprinkle pork chops with the remaining salt and cook, flipping once, until both sides are tender and heated through.
8. Transfer pork chops to a clean cutting board and chop crosswise.
9. Mix barbecue sauce and water in a pan and add the pork chops; turn to coat with the sauce.
10. Serve with kale and potatoes; drizzle with the remaining sauce in the pan.

Nutritional Information	Per Serving
Sodium	538 milligrams
Calories	364 milligrams
Fats	13 grams
Saturated Fats	2 grams
Dietary Fibers	4 grams
Carbohydrates	41 grams
Proteins	22 grams
Folates	38 micrograms
Cholesterol	57 milligrams
Sugar	7 grams
Vitamin C	31 milligrams
Calcium	62 milligrams
Iron	2 milligrams
Potassium	914 milligrams

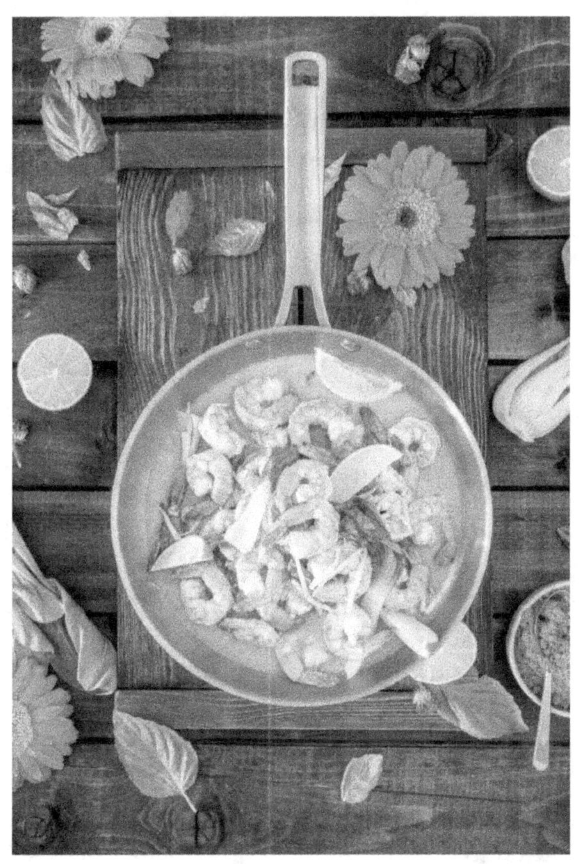

Orange Sesame Shrimp

Preparation 20 minutes   *Servings* 1
Nutritional Information
Shrimp is rich in proteins, plus it is high in multivitamins and minerals! In this DASH lunch recipe, shrimp is not only orange in color but taste like the orange fruit as well! Here's how:

Ingredients
½ piece ripe avocado
¼ cup orange juice extract

¼ cup apple cider vinegar
1 ½ cup finely sliced red cabbage
1 teaspoon sesame oil, toasted
2 tablespoons sugar
2 cup chopped romaine lettuce
2 tablespoons reduced sodium, gluten-free soy sauce
3 ounces peeled, cooked shrimp

Preparation

1. In a bowl, mix the orange juice extract, oil, vinegar, soy sauce, and sugar until the sugar has dissolved.
2. In another bowl, toss lettuce and cabbage to coat using the orange juice mixture.
3. Transfer to a serving platter and top it with shrimp and avocado.
4. Serve immediately.

Nutritional Information	Per Serving
Sodium	434 milligrams
Calories	283 milligrams
Fats	13 grams
Saturated Fats	2 grams
Fibers	9 grams
Carbohydrates	25 grams
Proteins	22 grams
Folates	239 micrograms
Cholesterol	137 milligrams
Sugar	13 grams
Vitamin A	8,578 international unit
Vitamin C	57 milligrams
Calcium	141 milligrams
Iron	3 milligrams
Potassium	1043 milligrams

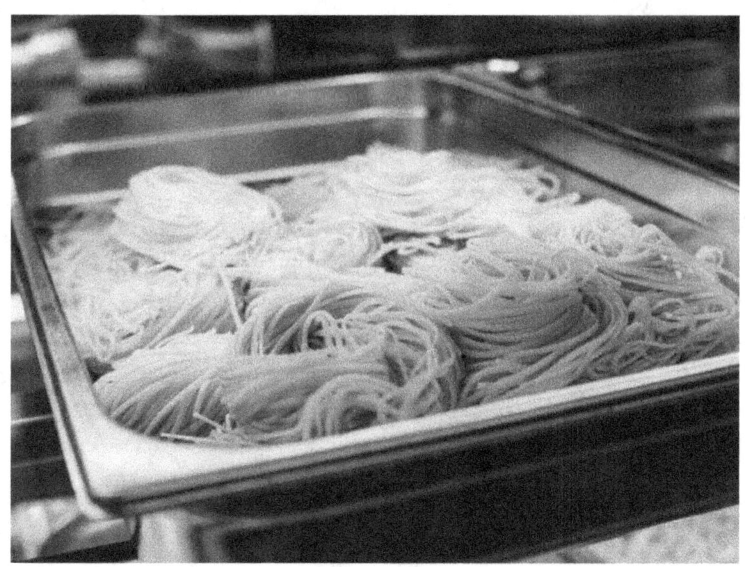

Creamy Chicken Pasta

Preparation 1-hour   *Servings* 4
Nutritional Information
Chicken is an excellent source of proteins, niacin, pantothenic acid, choline, selenium, B vitamins, and much more! Let me teach you how to cook a creamy pasta with chicken in the DASH diet way:

Ingredients
½ pack of angel hair pasta, whole wheat
½ teaspoon minced garlic
½ teaspoon iodized salt
½ teaspoon ground black pepper
½ cup water
¼ cup all-purpose flour
¼ cup reduced fat sour cream
1 shallot, large, finely sliced
2 tablespoons Dijon mustard
3 tablespoons sage
3 tablespoons extra-virgin olive oil
4 thinly sliced chicken breast cutlets

Preparation
1. In a saucepan, bring water to a boil to cook the angel hair pasta; drain completely.
2. In a bowl, coat chicken breast cutlets with flour, garlic, salt and pepper.
3. In a skillet, war, canola oil over medium-high heat to cook the chicken breast cutlets, flipping once, until golden brown and heated through for about 5 minutes on each side; transfer to a serving dish.
4. Reduce heat to medium then add the remaining oil to the saucepan to cook the shallot. Cook and stir frequently until it turns brownish; add the remaining flour mixture in water and cook until the consistency thickens.
5. Remove from heat then stir in the sour cream, mustard, sage, and the remaining salt and pepper.
6. Return chicken to the saucepan and turn it to coat with the creamy sauce.
7. Top the angel hair pasta with half of the creamy sauce.
8. Garnish with sage and serve.

Nutritional Information	Per Serving
Sodium	463 milligrams
Calories	447 milligrams
Fats	16 grams
Saturated Fats	3 grams
Fibers	6 grams
Carbohydrates	42 grams
Proteins	31 grams
Folates	41 micrograms
Cholesterol	68 milligrams
Sugar	2 grams
Vitamin A	154 international unit
Vitamin C	1 milligram
Calcium	60 milligrams
Iron	3 milligrams
Potassium	367 milligrams

DASH Meaty Spaghetti

Preparation 1-hour   *Servings* 8
Nutritional Information
Cook and serve a meaty spaghetti during parties and other celebrations in the DASH diet way. Here's how to make this recipe:

Ingredients

½ teaspoon iodized salt
½ cup grated Parmesan cheese
¼ cup coarsely chopped flat leaf parsley
1 pound whole wheat spaghetti
1 large finely chopped onion
1 large cubed carrot
1 stalk of minced celery
1 tablespoon Italian seasoning
1 pound 90% lean ground beef
1 can (28 ounces) crushed tomatoes
2 teaspoons extra-virgin olive oil
4 minced garlic cloves

Preparation

1. In a pot, bring water to a boil to cook the spaghetti; drain completely.
2. In a skillet, heat extra-virgin olive oil over medium heat to cook the carrots, onions, and celery; stir frequently until the onion turns translucent.
3. Add the garlic and Italian seasoning and cook until it smells fragrant.
4. Add the ground beef and stir to break it to bite-sized, cook until it turns brown.
5. Increase to high heat and add the tomatoes; cook until the consistency of the sauce thickens.
6. Add parsley and a dash more salt.

7. Transfer the meaty spaghetti to a serving bowl; pour sauce over the pasta and sprinkle with cheese.

Nutritional Information	Per Serving
Sodium	484 milligrams
Calories	389 milligrams
Fats	9 grams
Carbohydrates	54 grams
Proteins	27 grams
Folates	55 micrograms
Cholesterol	48 milligrams
Sugar	8 grams
Vitamin A	1,946 international unit
Vitamin C	14 milligrams
Calcium	120 milligrams
Iron	5 milligrams
Potassium	711 milligrams

Pork Chop Curry with Roasted Apples and Leeks

Preparation 1-hour   *Servings* 4

Nutritional Information

Pork is rich in meat proteins, amino acids, vitamins, and minerals. It is served with apples, which are rich in antioxidants, flavonoids, phytonutrients, dietary fibers, vitamins C and B; leeks are an excellent source of vitamin K, omega-3 fatty acids, carotenoids, calcium, magnesium, and much more!

Ingredients

½ teaspoon iodized salt

½ teaspoon ground black pepper

1 tablespoon cider vinegar

1 tablespoon brown sugar

1 tablespoon curry powder

1 large leek, halved lengthwise, including the white and light green parts, cleaned thoroughly

3 red apples, large, sliced thinly

3 tablespoons extra-virgin olive oil

4 pieces of pork chops, chopped into ½ to ¾ inch thick pieces

Preparation

1. In the oven, position the grill racks in the upper and lower third part; preheat to 425 °F.
2. Coat 2 rimmed baking sheets with extra-virgin olive oil.
3. In a bowl, combine extra-virgin olive oil, apples and leeks, then season with salt and pepper. Spread contents onto a baking sheet, then put it in the preheated oven (lower grill rack) and stir frequently for about 20 minutes until the apples are light brownish and the leeks are wilted.
4. Mix the curry powder in the used bowl and use it to coat the pork chops; allow to sit until the apples and leeks are done.
5. Leave the apples and leeks mixture in the oven; turn the broiler on high heat.

6. Place the pork chops on the upper grill rack and broil until an instant-read internal thermometer registers 145 °F.

7. In another bowl, mix the brown sugar and vinegar together until the sugar dissolves; add in the apples and leeks mixture, toss to combine.

8. Put the mixture on a serving platter, then add the pork chops and serve immediately.

Nutritional Information	Per Serving
Sodium	365 milligrams
Calories	429 milligrams
Fats	20 grams
Saturated Fats	4 grams
Dietary Fibers	5 grams
Carbohydrates	31 grams
Proteins	33 grams
Folates	20 micrograms
Cholesterol	100 milligrams
Vitamin A	463 international unit
Vitamin C	10 milligrams
Calcium	63 milligrams
Iron	2 milligrams
Potassium	672 milligrams

Roasted Pork Tenderloin with Rhubarb Barbecue Sauce

Preparation 1-hour   *Servings* 4

Nutritional Information

Pork is high in meat proteins and other essential vitamins, minerals, and amino acids, while rhubarb is a good source of fibers and vitamin K. Combine the two ingredients and infuse with barbecue for the flavorful DASH lunch recipe below:

Ingredients

½ teaspoon ground black pepper
¼ cup ketchup
¼ cup light brown sugar
¼ teaspoon iodized salt
1 tablespoon cider vinegar
1 small, minced onion
1 (1 pound) pork tenderloin slab, trimmed
2 teaspoons Worcestershire sauce
2 minced garlic cloves
2 cups frozen, thawed, minced Rhubarb
2 tablespoons extra-virgin olive oil

Preparation

1. Preheat oven to 425 °F.
2. In a saucepan, cook the garlic and onions in extra-virgin olive oil over medium heat; stir until it softens for a few minutes.
3. Add and stir the rhubarb, Worcestershire sauce, and ground black pepper together.
4. Bring to a simmer and cook for about 10 minutes, stirring frequently until the onions are translucent and the rhubarbs are tender. Continue to cook covered; remove from heat after a few minutes.
5. Heat the remaining extra-virgin olive oil in an oven-proof skillet at medium-high temperature.

6. Season pork with salt and pepper then put it in the skillet and cook until brownish; transfer the skillet to the oven to roast the pork chops until an instant-read thermometer inserted in its thickest part reaches 145 °F.

7. Transfer the pork chops to a cutting board and allow to sit for a few minutes.

8. Slice thinly and serve on a platter with rhubarb barbecue sauce.

Nutritional Information	Per Serving
Sodium	395 milligrams
Calories	286 milligrams
Fats	10 grams
Saturated Fats	2 grams
Fibers	2 grams
Carbohydrates	25 grams
Proteins	25 grams
Folates	11 micrograms
Cholesterol	74 milligrams
Vitamin A	156 international unit
Vitamin C	8 milligrams
Calcium	86 milligrams
Iron	2 milligrams
Potassium	770 milligrams

Tuna Melts

Preparation 15 minutes   *Servings* 6

Nutritional Information

Tuna is a good source of omega-3 fatty acids, high-quality proteins, selenium, and vitamin D.

Ingredients

Dash of iodized salt

Dash of ground black pepper

¼ cup onion, minced

¼ cup organic, low-fat salad dressing

1/3 cup minced celery

2 pieces of split, whole-wheat English muffins

3 ounces reduced fat, grated cheddar cheese

6 ounces tuna fish, drained

Preparation

1. Preheat broiler.
2. In a bowl, combine the tuna fish, salad dressing, celery, and onion; season with salt and pepper.
3. Toast English muffin halves in a toaster oven.
4. Place the English muffin halves split side up on a baking sheet and top each with ¼ of the tuna mixture.
5. Put it in the preheated broiler and broil for a few minutes until heated through.
6. Open broiler to sprinkle cheese, then continue broiling until the cheese melts.
7. Remove from the broiler and serve on a platter with or without rice.

Nutritional Information	Per Serving
Sodium	417 milligrams
Calories	210 milligrams
Total Fats	6 grams
Carbohydrates	20 grams
Proteins	19 grams
Dietary Fibers	3 grams

Quinoa Meatless Balls

Preparation 15 minutes   *Servings* 24
Nutritional Information
Quinoa is gluten-free, rich in proteins, B vitamins, and antioxidants. It contains all the nine essential amino acids that the body needs, and much more! This DASH lunch recipe helps treat high blood pressure and other heart-related diseases.

Ingredients
½ teaspoon sea salt
1/3 cup parmesan grated cheese
1/3 cup chives
1 ¾ cup whole grain breadcrumbs
1 tablespoon extra-virgin olive oil
1 piece of small minced onion
2 ½ cup cooked Quinoa
3 garlic cloves
4 eggs

Preparation
1. In a bowl, mix all the ingredients above
2. Mold the mixture into balls
3. Grease a skillet with extra-virgin olive oil
4. Cook the quinoa balls until brownish for about 10 minutes

Nutritional Information	Per Serving
Sodium	0 milligrams
Calories	120 milligrams
Carbohydrates	21 grams
Proteins	4 grams
Fats	1 gram
Fibers	2 grams

Quinoa Black Bean Burger

Preparation 1-hour   *Servings* 5

Nutritional Information

Quinoa is gluten-free, rich in proteins, B vitamins, and antioxidants; it contains all the nine essential amino acids that the body needs, and much more. Black beans are a great source of molybdenum, a mineral that brings health benefits to the heart and body. Here's how to make this unique black burger.

Ingredients

½ cup water
½ cup breadcrumbs
½ teaspoon iodized salt
¼ cup minced yellow bell pepper
¼ cup quinoa
1 piece of egg
1 ½ teaspoon ground cumin
1 large garlic clove, minced
1 can (15 ounces) black beans, rinsed and drained
2 tablespoons minced onion
3 tablespoons olive oil
5 whole wheat burger buns

Preparation

1. In a saucepan, bring the quinoa and water to a boil; once it bubbles, reduce the heat to simmer covered for about 15-20 minutes until the water is absorbed by the quinoa.
2. With a stainless-steel fork, mash the black beans to a paste.
3. In a bowl, mix the quinoa, black bean paste, onion, cumin, breadcrumbs, egg, garlic, salt, and pepper; form the black bean mixture into burger patties.
4. Heat olive oil in a skillet to cook the black bean burger patties; cook for a few minutes on each side.
5. Sandwich the black bean patty in the whole wheat burger buns.
6. Serve immediately.

Nutritional Information	Per Serving
Sodium	679 milligrams
Calories	245 milligrams
Fats	10 grams
Carbohydrates	28 grams
Proteins	9 grams
Cholesterol	37 grams

Cranberry Chicken Bowl

Preparation 30 minutes   *Servings* 12

Nutritional Information

Cranberries are an excellent source of manganese, vitamins C and E; chicken is rich in meat proteins, selenium, and antioxidants. This DASH lunch recipe is "berry" nutritious.

Ingredients

Dash of ground black pepper

½ cup minced green bell pepper

1 ½ cup dried cranberries

1 teaspoon iodized salt

1 cup coarsely chopped pecans

1 cup low-fat mayonnaise

1 teaspoon paprika

1 cup minced celery

2 green onions, minced

4 cups cubed, cooked chicken cutlets

Preparation

1. Mix all the ingredients in a bowl until blended well.
2. Refrigerate for 1-hour.
3. Remove from the refrigerator and reheat in a microwave oven.
4. Serve on a platter immediately.

Nutritional Information	Per Serving
Sodium	213 milligrams
Calories	315 milligrams
Fats	23 grams
Carbohydrates	15 grams
Proteins	13 grams
Cholesterol	42 milligrams

Chapter 6 – A Dash of Delectable Desserts

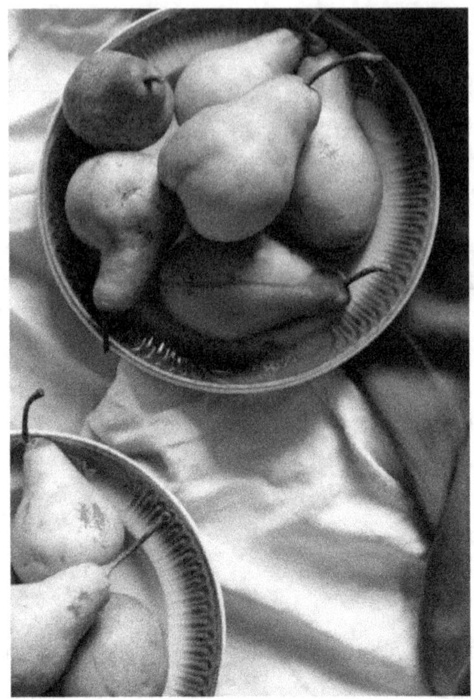

Poached Pears

Preparation 30 minutes   *Servings* 4

Nutritional Information

Pears are rich in antioxidants, dietary fibers, and much more!

Ingredients

¼ cup apple juice extract

½ cup fresh raspberries

1 cup orange juice extract

1 teaspoon cinnamon, ground

1 teaspoon ground nutmeg

2 tablespoons orange zest

4 whole pears, peeled, destemmed, core removed

Preparation

1. In a bowl, combine the fruit juices, nutmeg, and cinnamon, and then stir evenly.

2. In a shallow pan, pour the fruit juice mixture, and set to medium fire.
3. After a few minutes, reduce the heat to simmer for 30 minutes; turn pears frequently to maintain poaching, do not boil.
4. Transfer poached pears to a serving bowl; garnish with orange zest and raspberries.

Nutritional Information	Per Serving
Total Fats	0.5 grams
Calories	140 grams
Proteins	1 grams
Total Carbohydrates	34 grams
Dietary Fibers	2 grams
Monounsaturated Fats	Trace
Saturated Fats	Trace
Sodium	9 milligrams

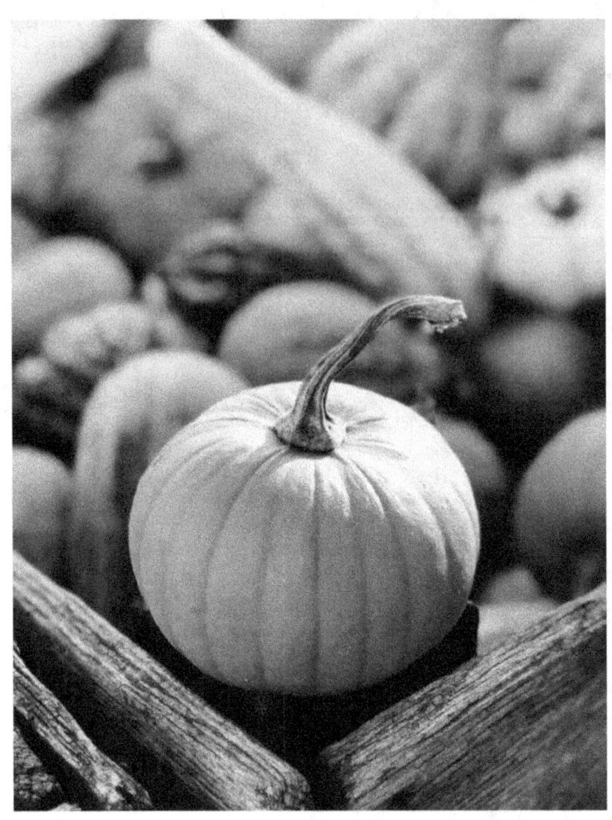

Pumpkin with Chia Seeds Pudding

Preparation 1-hour and 10 minutes   *Servings* 4
Nutritional Information
Pumpkin is a heart-healthy fruit which is rich in vitamin C, potassium, and fibers; chia seeds are highly concentrated with omega-3 fatty acids, antioxidants, fibers, calcium, and much more! Put the two ingredients to create a DASH pudding by following this recipe:

Ingredients for the Pudding
½ cup organic chia seeds
¼ cup raw maple syrup
1 ¼ cup low-fate milk

1 cup pumpkin puree extract

Ingredients for the Toppings
¼ cup organic sunflower seeds
¼ cup coarsely chopped almonds
¼ cup blueberries

Preparation
1. Add all the ingredients for the pudding in a bowl and mix until blended.
2. Cover and store in a chiller for 1-hour.
3. Remove from the chiller, transfer contents to a jar and add the ingredients for the toppings.
4. Serve immediately.

Nutritional Information	Per Serving
Sodium	42 milligrams
Calories	189 milligrams
Total Fats	7 grams
Saturated Fats	1 gram
Cholesterol	6 milligrams
Potassium	311 milligrams
Total Carbohydrates	27 grams
Dietary Fibers	4 grams
Proteins	5 grams
Sugar	18 grams

DASH Chocolate Truffles

Preparation 20 minutes   *Servings* 24
Nutritional Information
If you thought eating chocolate truffles is strictly prohibited in the DASH diet, think again! There is actually a DASH diet version and here is the recipe:

Ingredients for the Truffles
½ cup cacao powder
¼ cup chia seeds
¼ cup flaxseed meal
¼ cup maple syrup
1 cup flour
2 tablespoons almond milk
Ingredients for the Coatings
Cacao powder
Chia seeds
Flour
Shredded coconut, unsweetened
Preparation
1. Place all the ingredients for the truffle in a blender; pulse together until it is fully blended; transfer contents to a bowl.
2. Form into chocolate balls, then cover with the coating ingredients.
3. Serve immediately or store in a container with a lid (good for up to 5 days).

Nutritional Information	Per Serving
Sodium	2 milligrams
Calories	70 milligrams
Total Fats	1 gram
Total Carbohydrates	14 grams
Dietary Fibers	2 grams
Sugar	11 grams
Proteins	1 gram

Grilled Pineapple Strips

Preparation 15 minutes   *Servings* 6

Nutritional Information

Pineapple is a great source of manganese, B vitamins, vitamin C, pantothenic acid, copper, fibers, folates, and much more! Here's how to make the simplest DASH dessert:

Ingredients

Vegetable oil

Dash of iodized salt

1 pineapple

1 tablespoon lime juice extract

1 tablespoon olive oil

1 tablespoon raw honey

3 tablespoons brown sugar

Preparation

1. Peel the pineapple, remove the eyes of the fruit, and discard the core.
2. Slice lengthwise, forming six wedges.
3. Mix the remaining ingredients in a bowl until blended.
4. Brush the coating mixture on the pineapple (reserve some for basting).
5. Grease an oven or outdoor grill rack with vegetable oil.
6. Place the pineapple wedges on the grill rack and heat for a few minutes per side until golden brownish ; basting it frequently with a reserved glaze.
7. Serve on a platter.

Nutritional Information	Per Serving
Calories	97 milligrams
Fats	2 grams
Cholesterol	0 milligrams
Saturated Fats	0 milligrams
Carbohydrates	20 grams
Sugar	17 grams
Fibers	1 gram
Proteins	1 gram

Raspberry Peach Pancake

Preparation 1-hour   *Servings* 4
Nutritional Information
Raspberries are rich in ellagic acid and gallic acid; peaches are rich in vitamin C and antioxidants. Combine the two delicious fruits in a DASH pancake by following this "berry" nutritious recipe below:

Ingredients
½ teaspoon sugar
½ cup raspberries
½ cup fat-free milk
½ cup all-purpose flour
¼ cup vanilla yogurt
1/8 teaspoon iodized salt
1 tablespoon butter
2 medium peeled, thinly sliced peaches
3 lightly beaten organic eggs

Preparation
1. Preheat oven to 400 °F.
2. Toss peaches and raspberries with sugar in a bowl.
3. Melt butter in a 9-inch round baking plate.
4. Whisk together eggs, milk, and salt together in a small bowl until blended; whisk in the flour.
5. Remove the round baking plate from the oven, tilt to coat the bottom and sides with the melted butter; pour in the flour mixture.
6. Put it in the oven until it becomes brownish and puffed.
7. Remove the pancake from the oven.
8. Serve immediately with more raspberries and vanilla yogurt.

Nutritional Information	Per Serving
Sodium	173 milligrams
Calories	199 milligrams
Fats	7 grams
Saturated Fats	3 grams
Cholesterol	149 milligrams
Carbohydrates	25 grams
Sugar	11 grams
Fibers	3 grams
Proteins	9 grams

Mango Rice Pudding

Preparation 1-hour   *Servings* 4

Nutritional Information

Mango is rich in pectin, vitamin C, and fibers; rice is a great source of vitamins and minerals. This is not your ordinary DASH dessert. Here's how to prepare this pudding:

Ingredients

½ teaspoon ground cinnamon
¼ teaspoon iodized salt
1 teaspoon vanilla extract
1 cup long grain uncooked brown rice
2 medium ripe, peeled, cored mango
1 cup vanilla soymilk
2 tablespoons sugar
2 cups of water

Preparation

1. Bring saltwater to a boil in a saucepan to cook rice; after a few minutes, reduce the heat and simmer covered for 30-35 minutes until the water is absorbed by the rice.
2. Mash the mango with a mortar and pestle or stainless-steel fork.
3. Pour milk, sugar, cinnamon, and the mashed mango into the rice; cook uncovered on low heat, stirring frequently until the liquid is fully absorbed.
4. Remove the mango rice pudding from the heat, then stir in the vanilla soymilk.
5. Serve immediately or refrigerate and serve chilled; add mango cubes on top if desired.

Nutritional Information	Per Serving
Sodium	176 milligrams
Calories	275 milligrams
Fats	3 grams
Saturated Fats	0 milligrams
Cholesterol	0 milligrams
Carbohydrates	58 milligrams

| Sugar | 20 grams |
| Fibers | 3 grams |

Choco Banana Cake

Preparation 1-hour   *Servings* 18
Nutritional Information
Surprisingly, chocolate help treat high blood pressure and contains almost all the essential nutrients your body needs, including proteins, calcium, magnesium, copper, and antioxidants. Bananas are filled with a variety of multivitamins and minerals.

Ingredients
½ cup semisweet dark chocolate
½ cup brown sugar
½ teaspoon baking soda
¼ cup unsweetened cocoa powder
¼ cup canola oil
¾ cup soymilk
1 large egg
1 egg white
1 large, ripe, mashed banana
1 tablespoon lemon juice extract
1 teaspoon vanilla extract
2 cups all-purpose flour

Preparation
1. Preheat the oven to 350 °F.
2. Coat a baking pan with a non-stick spray.
3. Whisk together brown sugar, flour, baking soda, and cocoa powder in a bowl.
4. In another bowl, whisk together bananas, lemon juice extract, vanilla extract, oil, soymilk, egg, and egg whites.
5. Make a hole in the center of the flour mixture, then pour in the banana mixture and mix in the dark chocolate.
6. Stir all the ingredients with a spoon until fully blended; spoon the batter onto the baking pan.
7. Place in the oven and bake for 25-30 minutes until the center springs back when pressed lightly using your fingertips.

Nutritional Information	Per Serving
Sodium	52 milligrams
Calories	150 milligrams
Cholesterol	12 milligrams
Carbohydrates	27 grams
Saturated Fats	1 gram
Proteins	3 grams

Zesty Zucchini Muffins

Preparation 30 minutes   *Servings* 12

Nutritional Information

Eating zucchini promotes a healthy heart, lowers blood sugar levels, and help treat hypertension. Lemon keeps you hydrated and promotes healthy weight loss and much more! Combine the two ingredients to create DASH muffins that you can munch on without any weight concerns; just follow the recipe below:

Ingredients

Vegetable oil cooking spray
½ cup sugar
¼ teaspoon iodized salt
¼ teaspoon ground nutmeg
¾ cup skim milk
1 cup shredded zucchini
1 tablespoon baking powder
1 large egg
2 teaspoons grated lemon rind
2 cups of all-purpose flour
3 tablespoons vegetable oil

Preparation

1. Mix the flour, baking powder, sugar, salt, and lemon rinds in a bowl.
2. Make a well in the center of the flour mixture.
3. In another bowl, mix zucchini, milk, vegetable oil, and egg.
4. Coat muffin cups with vegetable oil cooking spray.
5. Divide the batter equally in 12 muffin cups.
6. Transfer the muffin cups to the baking pan and put it in a microwave oven and bake at 400 °F for 30 minutes until light golden brown.
7. Remove from the baking pan and allow to cool on a wire rack before serving.

Nutritional Information	Per Serving
Sodium	211.5 milligrams
Calories	169 milligrams
Total Fats	4.8 grams
Saturated Fats	0.4 gram
Polyunsaturated Fats	1.3 gram
Monounsaturated Fats	2.6 grams
Cholesterol	0.1 gram
Potassium	80.2 grams
Total Carbohydrates	29.1 grams
Dietary Fibers	2.5 grams
Sugar	12.8 grams

Blueberry Oat Muffins

Preparation 35 minutes   *Servings* 12

Nutritional Information

Blueberries help wash away cholesterol in the bloodstream and help reduce the risk of heart diseases; oats help lower the cholesterol levels and stabilize blood sugar (glucose) levels.

Ingredients

½ cup raw oatmeal
½ teaspoon baking powder
½ teaspoon iodized salt
½ cup dry milk
¼ cup vegetable oil
¼ teaspoon baking soda
1/3 cup sugar
1 ½ cup flour
1 cup milk
1 cup blueberries

Preparation

1. Preheat oven to 350 °F.
2. Coat the muffin tins with vegetable oil.
3. In a bowl, mix the flour, baking powder, baking soda, oats, sugar, and salt.
4. Mix milk, dry milk, egg, and vegetable oil in another bowl.
5. Pour the bowl of wet ingredients into the bowl of dry ingredients and mix partially.
6. Add the blueberries and mix until the consistency turns lumpy.
7. Scoop blueberry batter into the muffin tins.
8. Put it in the preheated oven and bake for 30 minutes until the muffins turn golden brown on the edges.
9. Serve warm immediately or put it in an airtight container and store in the refrigerator to serve chilled.

Nutritional Information	Per Serving
Sodium	180 milligrams
Calories	150 milligrams
Fats	5 grams
Saturated Fats	0.5 gram
Carbohydrates	22 grams
Proteins	4 grams
Fibers	1 gram

DASH Banana Bread

Preparation 1-hour and 10 minutes   *Servings* 14
Nutritional Information

Bananas bring your body a lot of multivitamins and minerals; these are an excellent source of magnesium and potassium. Here is the recipe to make the DASH version of your favorite banana bread:

Ingredients

Vegetable oil cooking spray
½ cup brown rice flour
½ cup amaranth flour
½ cup tapioca flour
½ cup millet flour
½ cup quinoa flour
½ cup raw sugar
¾ cup egg whites
1/8 teaspoon iodized salt
1 teaspoon baking soda
2 tablespoons grapeseed oil
2 pieces of mashed banana

Preparation

1. Preheat oven to 350 °F.
2. Coat a loaf pan with a vegetable oil cooking spray, dust evenly with a bit of flour and set aside.
3. In a bowl, mix the brown rice flour, amaranth flour, tapioca flour, millet flour, quinoa flour, and baking soda.
4. Coat a separate bowl with vegetable oil, then mix eggs, sugar, and mashed bananas.
5. Pour the bowl of wet ingredients into the bowl of dry ingredients and mix thoroughly.
6. Scoop the mixture into the loaf pan.
7. Put it in the preheated oven and bake for an hour.

8. To check the doneness, insert a toothpick in the center of the loaf pan; if you remove the toothpick and it has no batter sticking to it, remove the bread from the oven.

9. Slice and serve immediately and store the remaining banana bread in a refrigerator to prolong shelf life.

Nutritional Information	Per Serving
Sodium	150 milligrams
Calories	150 milligrams
Total Fats	3 grams
Fibers	2 grams
Proteins	4 grams
Sugar	7 grams

DASH Milk Chocolate Pudding

Preparation 1-hour and 15 minutes   *Servings* 4

Nutritional Information

Did you know that eating milk chocolate pudding is actually good for the heart? Milk chocolate is scientifically proven to help reduce the risks of heart diseases! Here's how to make the DASH version of everyone's favorite milk chocolate pudding:

Ingredients

½ teaspoon vanilla extract

1/3 cup chocolate chips

1/8 teaspoon salt

2 cups non-fat milk

2 tablespoons cocoa powder

2 tablespoons sugar

3 tablespoons cornstarch

Preparation

1. Mix cocoa powder, cornstarch, sugar, and salt in a saucepan and whisk in milk; stir frequently over medium heat until the pudding thickens and begins to bubble.
2. Remove from heat, then add the chocolate chips and vanilla extract; stir until the chocolate chips and vanilla melt into the pudding.
3. Pour contents into serving bowls and store in a chiller.
4. Serve chilled.

Nutritional Information	Per Serving
Sodium	5 milligrams
Calories	197 milligrams
Total Fats	5 grams
Saturated Fats	2.5 grams
Cholesterol	0 milligrams
Total Carbohydrates	9 grams
Dietary Fibers	0 gram
Proteins	0.5 gram

Minty Lime and Grapefruit Yogurt Parfait

Preparation 15 minutes   *Servings* 6

Nutritional Information

Grapefruit is an excellent source of vitamin A in the form of carotenoids, pantothenic acid, phytochemicals such as lycopene, antioxidants, and much more; lime helps reduce the risk of heart diseases and help lower blood sugar (glucose) levels; mint will make your DASH dessert literally "cool."

Ingredients

A handful of torn mint leaves

2 teaspoons grated lime zest

2 tablespoons lime juice extract

3 tablespoons raw honey

4 large red grapefruits

4 cups reduced fat plain yogurt

Preparation

1. Slice the top and bottom part of the red grapefruits and stand the fruit upright on a cutting board. Remove the peel with a knife and slice along the membrane of each segment to remove the skin.
2. Mix yogurt, lime juice extract, and lime zest in a bowl.
3. Layer half of the grapefruit and yogurt mixture into 6 parfait glasses; add another layer until the glass is filled and then drizzle with honey and top with mint leaves.
4. Serve immediately.

Nutritional Information	Per Serving
Sodium	115 milligrams
Calories	207 milligrams
Fats	3 grams
Saturated Fats	2 grams
Cholesterol	10 milligrams
Carbohydrates	39 milligrams
Sugar	36 grams
Fibers	3 grams

DASH Peach Tarts

Preparation 1-hour + cooling time   *Servings* 8

Nutritional Information

Peaches help lower cholesterol levels, making you feel energized the whole day.

Tart Ingredients

¼ cup softened butter

¼ teaspoon ground nutmeg

1 cup all-purpose flour

3 tablespoons sugar

Filling Ingredients

¼ teaspoon ground cinnamon

¼ cup coarsely chopped almonds

1/8 teaspoon almond extract

1/3 cup sugar

2 pounds medium, peeled, thinly sliced peaches

Preparation

1. Preheat oven to 375 °F.
2. Mix butter, nutmeg, and sugar in a bowl until light and fluffy.
3. Add and beat in flour until well-blended.
4. Place the batter on an ungreased fluted tart baking pan and press firmly on the bottom and top sides.
5. Put it in the medium rack of the preheated oven and bake for about 10 minutes until it turns to a crust.
6. In a bowl, coat peaches with sugar, flour, cinnamon, almond extract, and almonds.
7. Open the oven and put the tart crust on the lower rack of the oven and pour in the peach filling; bake for about 40-45 minutes.
8. Once done, remove from the oven, allow to cool, and serve; or cover with a cling wrap and refrigerate to serve chilled.

Nutritional Information	Per Serving
Sodium	46 milligrams
Calories	222 milligrams
Fats	8 grams
Saturated Fats	4 grams
Cholesterol	15 milligrams
Carbohydrates	36 grams
Sugar	21 grams
Fibers	3 grams
Proteins	4 grams

DASH Raspberry Nuts Parfait

Preparation 10 minutes   *Servings* 1

Nutritional Information

Raspberries are rich in ellagic acid; nuts such as almonds are filled with healthy fats that help reduce hunger pangs, promoting healthy weight loss, reducing the risk of high blood pressure and lowering blood sugar (glucose) levels.

Ingredients

¼ cup frozen raspberries

¼ cup frozen blueberries

¼ cup toasted, thinly sliced almonds

1 cup non-fat, plain Greek yogurt

2 teaspoons raw honey

Preparation

1. First, layer Greek yogurt in a parfait glass; add berries; layer yogurt again, top with almonds and more berries; drizzle with honey.
2. Serve chilled.

Nutritional Information	Per Serving
Sodium	83 milligrams
Calories	378 milligrams
Fats	15 grams
Saturated Fats	1 gram
Fibers	6 grams
Carbohydrates	35 grams
Proteins	30 grams
Folates	37 micrograms
Cholesterol	11 milligrams
Sugar	25 grams
Added Sugar	12 grams
Calcium	336 milligrams
Iron	2 milligrams
Potassium	610 milligrams

Strawberry Bruschetta

Preparation 30 minutes   *Servings* 20

Nutritional Information

Strawberries are rich in phytonutrients, fibers, and vitamins C and K.

Ingredients

1 loaf sliced Ciabatta bread
8 ounces goat cheese
1 cup basil leaves
2 containers of strawberries, sliced
5 tablespoons balsamic glaze

Preparation

1. Wash and slice strawberries; set aside.
2. Wash and chop the basil leaves; set aside.
3. Slice the ciabatta bread and spread some goat cheese evenly on each slice; add strawberries, balsamic glaze, and top with basil leaves.
4. Serve on a platter.

Nutritional Information	Per Serving
Sodium	59 milligrams
Calories	80 milligrams
Fats	2 grams
Carbohydrates	12 grams
Proteins	3 grams

Chapter 7 – A Dash of Delicious Dinners

Wrap up the day by preparing and cooking the most delicious dinner for yourself and your family!

Black Beans and Sweet Potato Rice Bowl

Preparation 30 minutes   *Servings* 4

Nutritional Information

Black beans are an excellent source of fibers and proteins; sweet potatoes are rich in beta-carotene and antioxidants. Mix the two to make a nutritious DASH diet rice bowl before you go to sleep. Here's how to do it:

Ingredients

Lime wedges, optional

¼ teaspoon garlic salt

¾ cup uncooked long grain rice

1 can (15 ounces) rinsed and drained black beans

1 ½ cup water

1 large peeled, diced sweet potato

1 medium thinly sliced red onion

3 tablespoons olive oil

4 cups chopped, destemmed kale

Preparation

1. Pour water, rice, and garlic salt in a saucepan, then bring to a boil over medium-high heat. After a few minutes, reduce the heat to simmer, covered until the rice fully absorbs the water. Once cooked, allow to sit for 5 minutes.

2. In a skillet, heat olive oil over medium-high heat to sauté the sweet potatoes until light golden brown; add onions and stir until they turn translucent; add kale and stir until wilted; add the black beans and stir until cooked thoroughly.

3. Add rice to the skillet and stir with the rest of the ingredients.

4. Serve on a platter with lime wedges.

Nutritional Information	Per Serving
Sodium	405 milligrams
Calories	435 milligrams
Fats	11 grams
Saturated Fats	2 grams
Cholesterol	0 milligrams
Carbohydrates	74 grams
Sugar	15 grams
Proteins	10 grams

DASH Cannellini Corn Pasta

Preparation 30 minutes   *Servings* 8
Nutritional Information

This unique cannellini corn pasta makes a very nutritious DASH dinner with ingredients freshly produced from the farm to your family's table.

Ingredients

½ cup minced red onion
½ cup part-skim ricotta cheese
½ teaspoon ground black pepper
¼ cup Parmesan grated cheese
1 can (15 ounces) of cannellini beans, rinsed and drained
1 cup kernel corn
1 tablespoon olive oil
2 tablespoons minced basil
2 cups cherry tomatoes, halved
3 cups baby spinach
3 minced garlic cloves
3 cups (12 ounces) uncooked whole wheat elbow macaroni

Preparation

1. Cook the pasta in a stockpot according to the product instructions.
2. Combine all the ingredients in a bowl; stir in cooked pasta until coated and well-seasoned.
3. Serve in a bowl.

Nutritional Information	Per Serving
Sodium	429 milligrams
Calories	275 milligrams
Fats	5 grams
Saturated Fats	1 gram
Cholesterol	7 milligrams

Carbohydrates	46 grams
Sugar	4 grams
Fibers	8 grams
Proteins	13 grams

Orange and Pistachio-Crusted Pork Tenderloin with Rice

Preparation 1-hour   *Servings* 4
Nutritional Information

Oranges are an excellent source of several multivitamins and minerals; pistachio washes away bad cholesterol and help treat high blood pressure. Tenderloin is a great source of riboflavin, potassium, zinc and much more. Pair it with brown rice, which is rich in fibrous bran, a carb-rich endosperm. Here's how to make this delicious DASH dinner recipe:

Ingredients
½ cup pearl barley
½ cup wild rice
½ teaspoon ground black pepper
¼ cup shelled, toasted pistachios
¾ teaspoon iodized salt
1 ½ pound green beans, trimmed
1 pound pork tenderloin, trimmed
2 teaspoons lemon zest
2 tablespoons extra-virgin olive oil
2 garlic cloves
3 tablespoons orange juice extract
3 cups of water

Preparation
1. In a saucepan, mix water, pearl barley, brown rice, and iodized salt together and bring to a boil, covered; after a few minutes, reduce the heat to simmer until the contents are tender and the water is fully absorbed.
2. Position the oven racks in the middle and at the bottom; preheat to 450 °F.
3. Pulse the pistachios and garlic in a blender.
4. On a clean, working surface, season pork tenderloin with salt and pepper.

5. In a skillet, heat olive oil over medium-high heat; cook the pork tenderloins until tender and chewy; remove from heat once cooked.
6. Brush the top of the pork tenderloin with orange juice extract; top it with the pistachio mixture.
7. Transfer the pan to the upper rack of the oven and roast the pork tenderloins; check with an instant-read thermometer, if the thermometer inserted in the middle of the pork reaches 145 °F, transfer it to a clean cutting board and allow to cool for a few minutes before slicing.
8. Toss green beans in a bowl to coat with olive oil, lemon zest, salt and pepper; transfer to a baking sheet, then roast on the lower grill rack until tender and crisp for about 10 minutes.
9. Serve the pork tenderloins on a platter with green beans and brown rice.

Nutritional Information	Per Serving
Sodium	550 milligrams
Calories	498 milligrams
Fats	15 grams
Saturated Fats	3 grams
Fibers	11 grams
Carbohydrates	62 grams
Proteins	32 grams
Folates	89 micrograms
Cholesterol	60 milligrams
Sugar	16 grams
Vitamin A	1,219 international unit
Vitamin C	23 milligrams
Calcium	99 milligrams
Iron	4 milligrams
Potassium	971 milligrams

Chickpea Curry

Preparation 30 minutes   *Servings* 6
Nutritional Information
Chickpeas are filled with fibers and promote healthy weight loss.

Ingredients
Cilantro for garnish
½ teaspoon ground turmeric
¾ teaspoon kosher salt
1 medium Serrano pepper sliced in thirds
1 medium yellow onion, sliced into rings
1 2-inch piece of peeled, coarsely chopped ginger
2 ¼ cups of diced tomatoes
2 teaspoons ground coriander
2 teaspoons ground cumin
2 (15 ounces) cans chickpeas, washed and drained
2 teaspoons garam masala
4 minced garlic cloves
6 tablespoons canola oil

Preparation
1. Mix Serrano pepper, ginger, onion, and garlic in a blender.
2. Heat oil in a saucepan over medium-high heat to sauté onions until translucent; add the ground coriander, cumin, and turmeric.
3. Pulse tomatoes in a blender, then transfer onto the saucepan and dash with iodized salt; reduce the heat to simmer, and stir frequently.
4. Add the chickpeas and garam masala; cook covered and stir occasionally.
5. Once done, transfer contents to a serving bowl and garnish with cilantro.

Nutritional Information	Per Serving
Sodium	354 milligrams
Calories	278 milligrams
Fats	15 grams
Saturated Fats	1 gram
Fibers	6 grams
Carbohydrates	30 grams
Proteins	6 grams
Folates	75 micrograms
Sugar	3 grams
Vitamin A	260 international unit
Vitamin C	18 milligrams
Calcium	65 milligrams
Iron	2 milligrams
Potassium	356 milligrams

Fried Chicken with Cauliflower Rice Bowl

Preparation 1-hour   *Servings* 4
Nutritional Information
Chicken is a great source of niacin, proteins, pantothenic acid, choline, selenium, and much more; cauliflower is rich in biotin, omega-3 fatty acids, carotenoids, antioxidants, and much more!

In this DASH dinner recipe, we will teach you how cauliflower can be a good substitute for rice:

Ingredients
½ cup red bell pepper, diced
1 cup trimmed, halved snow peas
1 teaspoon vegetable oil
1 tablespoon grated ginger
1 tablespoon minced garlic
1 pound boneless, skinless chicken thighs, trimmed and chopped to bite-sized
2 large beaten eggs
3 scallions, sliced thinly, white and green parts separated
3 tablespoons gluten-free, low-sodium soy sauce
4 cups of cauliflower florets, crumbled

Preparation
1. In a skillet, heat vegetable oil on high to cook scrambled eggs; once cooked, transfer to a cutting board and slice into thin strips.
2. Heat vegetable oil in a saucepan to cook scallion whites, ginger, and garlic; once the scallions are soft and tender, add the chicken and then cook, stirring frequently, until it is light brownish and tender.
3. Add snow peas and red bell pepper, cook and stir frequently until tender.
4. Transfer everything to a large serving bowl.
5. Add the remaining vegetable oil to the pan to cook the crumbled cauliflower florets; stir to soften.

6. Put the chicken mixture in the saucepan and add eggs; pour soy sauce and mix well until combined.
7. Serve and garnish with scallion greens.

Nutritional Information	Per Serving
Sodium	591 milligrams
Calories	304 milligrams
Fats	15 grams
Saturated Fats	4 grams
Fibers	4 grams
Carbohydrates	12 grams
Proteins	30 grams
Folates	124 micrograms
Cholesterol	200 milligrams
Sugar	5 grams
Vitamin A	1,060 international unit
Vitamin C	108 milligrams
Calcium	75 milligrams
Iron	3 milligrams
Potassium	883 milligrams

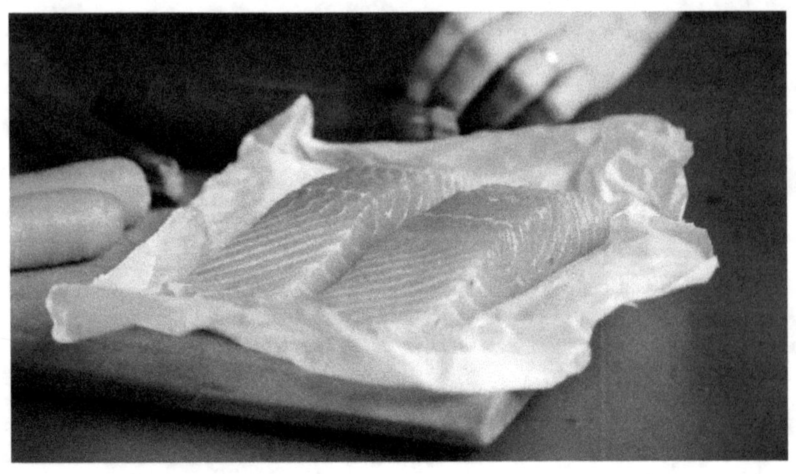

Garlic-Roasted Salmon with Brussel Sprouts

Preparation 1-hour   *Servings* 6
Nutritional Information
Salmon is an excellent source of omega-3 fatty acids, protein, niacin, and much more. Brussel sprouts are rich in glucosinolates. Combine the two ingredients into a DASH dinner by following the recipe below:

Ingredients
Lemon wedges
¼ cup extra-virgin olive oil
¾ teaspoon ground black pepper
¾ cup white wine; we highly recommend Chardonnay
1 teaspoon iodized salt
2 pounds of wild-caught salmon fillet, skin on, sliced in 6 portions
2 tablespoons finely sliced oregano
6 cups trimmed sliced Brussel sprouts
14 minced garlic cloves

Preparation
1. Preheat oven to 450 °F.
2. Toss oil, garlic, oregano, salt, and pepper in a bowl.

3. Halve the garlic mixture and toss Brussel sprouts and seasoned oil, then transfer contents to a roasting pan.
4. Place in the preheated oven to roast; open once to stir.
5. Pour white wine into the remaining oil mixture.
6. Remove the pan from the oven, then stir the vegetables; top with salmon, drizzle with white wine, sprinkle with the remaining oregano; dash on salt and pepper.
7. Return to the oven and bake until the salmon is cooked thoroughly.
8. Once done, remove from the oven and serve on a platter with lemon wedges.

Nutritional Information	Per Serving
Sodium	485 milligrams
Calories	334 milligrams
Fats	15 grams
Saturated Fats	3 grams
Fibers	3 grams
Carbohydrates	10 grams
Proteins	33 grams
Folates	75 micrograms
Cholesterol	71 milligrams
Sugar	2 grams
Vitamin A	990 international unit
Vitamin C	64 milligrams
Calcium	115 milligrams
Iron	2 milligrams
Potassium	921 milligrams

Pork Curry with Rice Noodles

Preparation 30 minutes   *Servings* 1

Nutritional Information

Serve a different kind of dinner with rice noodles! Pork curry with rice noodles is a healthier alternative to regular noodles.

Ingredients

1 teaspoon brown sugar

1 cup chopped green beans

1 cup red shredded cabbage

2 tablespoons gluten-free, low-sodium soy sauce

2 tablespoons curry paste

2 minced garlic cloves

2 chopped scallions

3 tablespoons chopped cilantro

3 tablespoons toasted sesame oil

8 ounces boneless cubed pork tenderloin

8 ounces rice noodles

Preparation

1. Cook rice noodles according to the product instructions.
2. Mix the scallions, ginger, garlic, and brown sugar in a saucepan and cook over medium heat until it starts to sizzle.
3. Remove from heat then stir in soy sauce and curry paste.
4. Add the rice noodles to the pork tenderloin, red cabbage, green beans, and cilantro; toss to combine.
5. Serve in a shallow bowl.

Nutritional Information	Per Serving
Sodium	487 milligrams
Calories	407 milligrams
Fats	12 grams
Saturated Fats	2 grams
Fibers	2 grams
Carbohydrates	57 grams

Proteins	16 grams
Folates	20 micrograms
Cholesterol	41 milligrams
Sugar	3 grams
Vitamin A	534 international unit
Vitamin C	15 milligrams
Calcium	51 milligrams
Iron	3 milligrams
Potassium	387 milligrams

Spiced Turkey in Lettuce Cups

Preparation 30 minutes   *Servings* 4

Nutritional Information

Turkey has lower cholesterol levels than any other meat; lettuce is rich in minerals. Here's how to make a DASH recipe that turns lettuce into healthy cups:

Ingredients

½ cup water chestnuts
½ cup brown rice
½ cup low sodium chicken broth
½ teaspoon iodized salt
½ cup minced cilantro
1 large grated carrot
1 pound 93% lean ground turkey
1 tablespoon minced ginger
1 large diced red bell pepper
1 (8 ounce) can rinsed, coarsely chopped water chestnuts
2 heads Boston lettuce, leaves separated
2 teaspoons sesame oil
2 tablespoons hoisin sauce

Preparation

1. Bring water to a boil in a saucepan to cook brown rice; reduce the heat to simmer rice until the water is fully absorbed by it.

2. Cook turkey and ginger over medium-high heat in a non-stick pan while crumbling it into bite-sized pieces using a stainless steel spoon.

3. Once the turkey is cooked, stir in the cooked brown rice.

4. Add bell pepper, hoisin sauce, water chestnuts, chicken broth, and salt; mix until thoroughly cooked.

5. Distribute lettuce leaves on a serving platter and scoop the
    turkey mixture onto each leaf equally; top with cilantro,
    carrots, and roll the lettuce leaves to form a cup.

Nutritional Information	Per Serving
Sodium	595 milligrams
Calories	276 milligrams
Fats	10 grams
Saturated Fats	2 grams
Fibers	4 grams
Carbohydrates	21 grams
Proteins	26 grams
Folates	90 micrograms
Cholesterol	65 milligrams
Sugar	6 grams
Vitamin A	7,275 international unit
Vitamin C	58 milligrams
Calcium	57 milligrams
Iron	5 milligrams
Potassium	677 milligrams

Noodle-Less Lasagna

Preparation 1-hour and 30 minutes   *Servings* 8
Nutritional Information
Have you ever heard of a noodle-less lasagna? If not, try this unique DASH dinner by following the recipe below:

Ingredients
Vegetable oil cooking spray
½ onion, minced
¼ teaspoon ground black pepper
1 cup shredded mozzarella cheese
1 large eggplant, sliced lengthwise to ¼-inch strips
1 large zucchini, sliced lengthwise to ¼-inch strips
1 teaspoon dried basil
1 cup part-skim ricotta cheese
1 large egg
2 minced garlic cloves
12 ounces sweet Italian sausage, casings removed
28 ounces crushed tomatoes

Preparation
1. Preheat oven to 400 °F.
2. Coat two baking sheets with vegetable oil cooking spray.
3. Arrange the eggplants and zucchini in a single layer on the greased baking sheets; place in the preheated oven and roast for 30 minutes.
4. Cook the Italian sausage in a saucepan and crack it using a stainless-steel spoon; cook until brownish.
5. Add onions and garlic, stirring frequently until the onions are translucent and the garlic is light golden brown.
6. Add tomatoes, basil, and oregano, then cook, stirring frequently until it bubbles; reduce the heat to simmer.
7. Combine ricotta cheese, egg, and ground black pepper in a bowl.

8. Spread tomato sauce in a baking dish, top with a layer of eggplant, add a dollop of ricotta cheese mixture, sprinkle with mozzarella cheese, layer half of the zucchini, and layer the eggplant crosswise; repeat the layering pattern until the baking dish is filled.
9. Put the baking pan in the preheated oven and bake for 30 minutes.
10. Garnish with basil and serve immediately.

Nutritional Information	Per Serving
Sodium	506 milligrams
Calories	279 milligrams
Fats	16 grams
Saturated Fats	7 grams
Fibers	4 grams
Carbohydrates	19 grams
Proteins	17 grams
Folates	34 micrograms
Cholesterol	69 milligrams
Sugar	7 grams
Vitamin A	1,192 international unit
Vitamin C	16 milligrams
Calcium	208 milligrams
Iron	4 milligrams
Potassium	599 milligrams

DASH Chicken Piccata

Preparation 40 minutes   *Servings* 4
Nutritional Information
Chicken piccata is an Italian dish made of chicken breast cutlets coated with flour and served with a delicious sauce.

Ingredients
½ cup parmesan grated cheese
½ cup cornmeal
1 ½ cup mixed green beans soaked in oil and vinegar
1 cup grapes
1 teaspoon lemon pepper
1 cup low sodium chicken broth
1 tablespoon olive oil
1 pound boneless chicken breast, skin on, chopped bite-sized
1 teaspoon dried basil
1 teaspoon dried oregano
1 pack of baby potatoes
1 tablespoon butter
2 tablespoon lemon juice extract

Preparation
1. Preheat oven to 400 °F.
2. Place the baby potatoes in a baking pan, coat with vegetable oil cooking spray and toss the green beans, grapes, lemon pepper, basil, and oregano; put it in the oven.
3. Pound chicken breasts with a meat mallet.
4. Dredge chicken breast cutlets in the cornmeal and lemon pepper mixture.
5. Heat vegetable oil in a skillet at medium-high.
6. Pour in lemon juice extract, chicken broth, and add chicken cutlets; once it bubbles, reduce the heat to simmer and then add butter.
7. Serve the chicken piccata and potatoes on a platter.

Nutritional Information	Per Serving
Sodium	590 milligrams
Calories	520 milligrams
Dietary Fibers	2.9 grams
Total Fats	12.3 grams
Saturated Fats	4.8 grams
Fats	20 grams
Cholesterol	75 milligrams

DASH Shepherd's Pie

Preparation 1-hour and 5 minutes   *Servings* 6

Nutritional Information

Shepherd's pie is not your typical pie; it is a comfort food loaded with vegetables.

Ingredients

Dash of ground black pepper

Vegetable oil cooking spray

½ cup low-fat milk

½ cup shredded cheddar cheese

¾ cup low sodium beef broth

1 pound lean ground beef

1 medium onion, minced

1 clove minced garlic

2 tablespoons flour

2 large, peeled, diced potatoes

4 cups of your favorite mixed vegetables

Preparation

1. Put the diced potatoes in a saucepan and pour in enough water to soak the potatoes and bring to a boil; after a few minutes, reduce the heat to simmer the potatoes until tender.
2. Once potatoes are cooked, drain the saucepan completely; using a stainless-steel fork, mash the potatoes then pour milk and set aside.
3. Preheat oven to 375 °F.
4. Heat vegetable oil in a skillet to cook the ground beef, garlic, and onion; pour in the flour and cook for a minute, stirring frequently.
5. Add vegetables and beef broth; cook and stir well for a few minutes until it bubbles.
6. Transfer the vegetable mixture to a baking dish; spread the potato mixture evenly over the veggie and meat mixture; sprinkle cheese on top.

7. Bake for 25-30 minutes until it bubbles.

8. Serve immediately.

Nutritional Information	Per Serving
Sodium	200 grams
Calories	320 milligrams
Total Fats	7 grams
Carbohydrates	39 grams
Proteins	24 grams
Fibers	5 grams

DASH Roasted Turkey

Preparation 4 hours and 20 minutes   *Servings*
Nutritional Information
Celebrate Thanksgiving in a healthier way by cooking a DASH diet version of the famous roasted turkey dish. Here's how to roast turkey following this diet's parameters:

Ingredients
Dash of ground black pepper
1 whole turkey (about 10++ pounds), frozen, thawed
1 medium peeled, finely sliced shallot
2 carrots, sliced bite-sized
2 minced yellow onions
2 celery stalks, minced
4 thinly-sliced garlic cloves
8 Roma tomatoes, halved

Preparation
1. Preheat oven to 400 °F.
2. Place shallots, garlic, and ground black pepper in a bowl; mix and set aside.
3. Arrange the carrots, onions, and celery in a baking pan and place it in the bottom of the roasting pan.
4. Remove the turkey from its packaging, then cut off the neck and reserve it for making the turkey stock; remove and discard the giblets and fatty tissues (inside the neck and body cavities).
5. Rinse the turkey inside out and pat dry with paper towels.
6. Place the turkey breast-side-up surrounded by vegetables in the roasting pan; tuck the wing tips behind and rub the turkey with the shallot mixture.
7. Place turkey in the middle of the oven and roast uncovered.
8. Put it in the preheated oven and bake for 30 minutes; reduce the heat to 325 °F. After 3 and a half hours, check

the doneness by piercing the breast part with an instant-read thermometer. The internal temperature should reach 170-175 °F.

9. While roasting the turkey in the oven, place the turkey neck in a saucepan and pour in 4 cups of water. Cook over medium-high heat, simmer covered for an hour; this stock can either be used as a gravy or as a base for turkey soup.

10. Remove the turkey from the roasting oven and transfer to a serving platter. With a slotted spoon, pick up the vegetables and arrange them around the turkey.

11. Cover the turkey and the surrounding vegetables tightly with aluminum foil and allow to sit for 30 minutes before slicing and/or serving.

Nutritional Information	Per Serving
Calories	250 milligrams
Carbohydrates	4 grams
Fats	6 grams
Proteins	45 grams
Fibers	1 gram

DASH Mac and Cheese

Preparation 1-hour   *Servings* 8
Nutritional Information
Make mac (macaroni) and cheese healthier by following this DASH dinner recipe below:

Ingredients
Dash of ground black pepper
Dash of iodized salt
¾ pound whole wheat elbow macaroni
1/3 cup reduced fat grated cheddar cheese
1 tablespoon thyme
1 teaspoon unsalted butter
2 teaspoon unsalted butter
2 cups breadcrumbs
2 teaspoons Dijon mustard
3 tablespoon all-purpose flour

Preparation
1. Preheat oven to 400 °F.
2. Coat a baking dish with butter.
3. Fill a pot with water and a dash of iodized salt to cook macaroni until it is firm when bitten.
4. In a pan, melt butter to sauté breadcrumbs and season with ground black pepper. Stir over medium heat until the crumbs turn golden brown ; allow to sit then pour 1/3 of the cheddar cheese and toss to combine.
5. Melt butter at a medium-low heat in a saucepan, then pour flour and stir for a few minutes; whisk in milk then bring to a boil, whisking constantly while simmering.
6. Add and stir in the remaining cheddar, Dijon mustard, thyme, and ground black pepper.
7. In a bowl, mix elbow macaroni, chicken stock, and turkey sauce; transfer to a baking dish.

8. Sprinkle the breadcrumbs and cheese mixture evenly over the elbow macaroni mixture and place it in the middle rack of the oven.

9. Bake for 25-30 minutes until it turns light golden brown.

Nutritional Information	Per Serving
Sodium	360 milligrams
Calories	350 milligrams
Total Fats	8 grams
Carbohydrates	54 grams
Proteins	19 grams
Fibers	6 grams

Lime Tilapia Fillets

Preparation 30 minutes   *Servings* 4
Nutritional Information
Tilapia is rich in potassium, niacin, selenium, phosphorus, vitamin B12, and much more; adding lime to your fillets help lower blood sugar (glucose) levels and help reduce the risk of high blood pressure. Here's how to make tilapia filets with a twist of DASH:

Ingredients
Lime wedges for garnish
Dash of iodized salt
Dash of ground black pepper
¼ cup coarsely chopped cilantro
1 medium avocado
1 pound tilapia fillets, washed and patted dry
1 teaspoon olive oil
1 small minced onion
1 cup shredded cabbage
2 pieces jalapeño peppers, sliced thinly, seeds removed
3 tablespoons lime juice extract
4 minced garlic cloves
4 tablespoons fat free sour cream
8 pieces (5-inch each) of white corn tortillas

Preparation
1. Heat olive oil in a skillet to sauté onions and garlic; cook until the onions are translucent and the garlic is light brown. Add the tilapia fillets to fry, flip once and cook until crispy on both side.
2. Pour the lime juice; add the jalapeño peppers, tomatoes, and cilantro; sauté over medium-high heat for a few minutes and break the tilapia fillets to mix everything well. Dash with salt and pepper to add more flavor.
3. Slice the avocado thinly on a cutting board and finely shred the cabbage.

4. Transfer tilapia fillets onto a serving plate, surround it with the avocados, cabbage shredding, cilantro, and lime wedges; serve with sour cream.

Nutritional Information	Per Serving
Sodium	142 milligrams
Calories	427 milligrams
Total Fats	12 grams
Saturated Fats	2 grams
Carbohydrates	45 grams
Proteins	35 grams
Fibers	5 grams
Calcium	60 milligrams

Beef Stroganoff

Preparation 1 hour   *Servings* 4

Nutritional Information

Eating beef for dinner is healthy for the heart; it is rich in iron, protein, zinc, and B vitamins.

Ingredients

Olive oil

½ cup onion, minced

½ pound beef round steak, boneless, sliced ¾-inch thick, all fat removed

½ can of fat-free cream of mushroom soup

½ cup water

½ teaspoon paprika

½ cup fat free sour cream

1 tablespoon all-purpose flour

4 cups of egg noodles, yolkless

Preparation

1. In a non-stick frying pan, heat olive oil to sauté onions over medium heat until they turn translucent.
2. Add the beef round steak and cook until brown and tender; drain completely and set aside.
3. Fill a pot with water that is enough to boil noodles until tender; drain completely and set aside.
4. In a saucepan, whisk together the cream of mushroom soup, water, and flour over medium heat; stir well until the consistency thickens.
5. Pour the soup mixture and the paprika onto the beef round steaks in the frying pan. Cook over medium heat and stir until heated through; remove from heat then add the sour cream and stir together to combine.
6. To serve, divide the pasta equally among the serving plates, then top it with the beef mixture.

Nutritional Information	Per Serving
Sodium	307 milligrams
Calories	302 milligrams
Total Fats	6 grams
Fibers	2 grams
Proteins	24 grams
Carbohydrates	38 grams

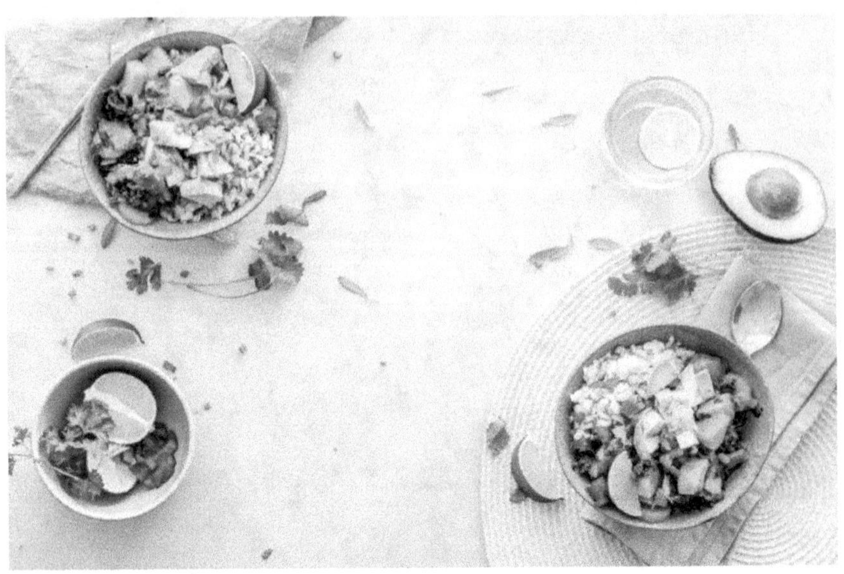

Conclusion

In the final analysis, the DASH diet, or the dietary approaches to stop hypertension, just like any other lifestyle interventions, promotes the optimal management of treating hypertension (also known as high blood pressure). This healthy eating approach can generally be implemented by most of the patient population and the results will never fail (especially your heart health!)

The DASH diet eating pattern comprises lean meat and seafood, green and leafy vegetables, citrus fruits, low-fat or fat-free dairy products, whole grains, unsweetened desserts, and DASH diet-infused beverages. It strongly and effectively helps lower blood pressure (BP) along with a combination of hospital treatments and prescription drugs.

What was your motivation for selecting this book? Please let me know your feedback and thoughts by **leaving a review on Amazon**, *because this 'open' way of communicating may help others who have read the book or are interested in reading it.*